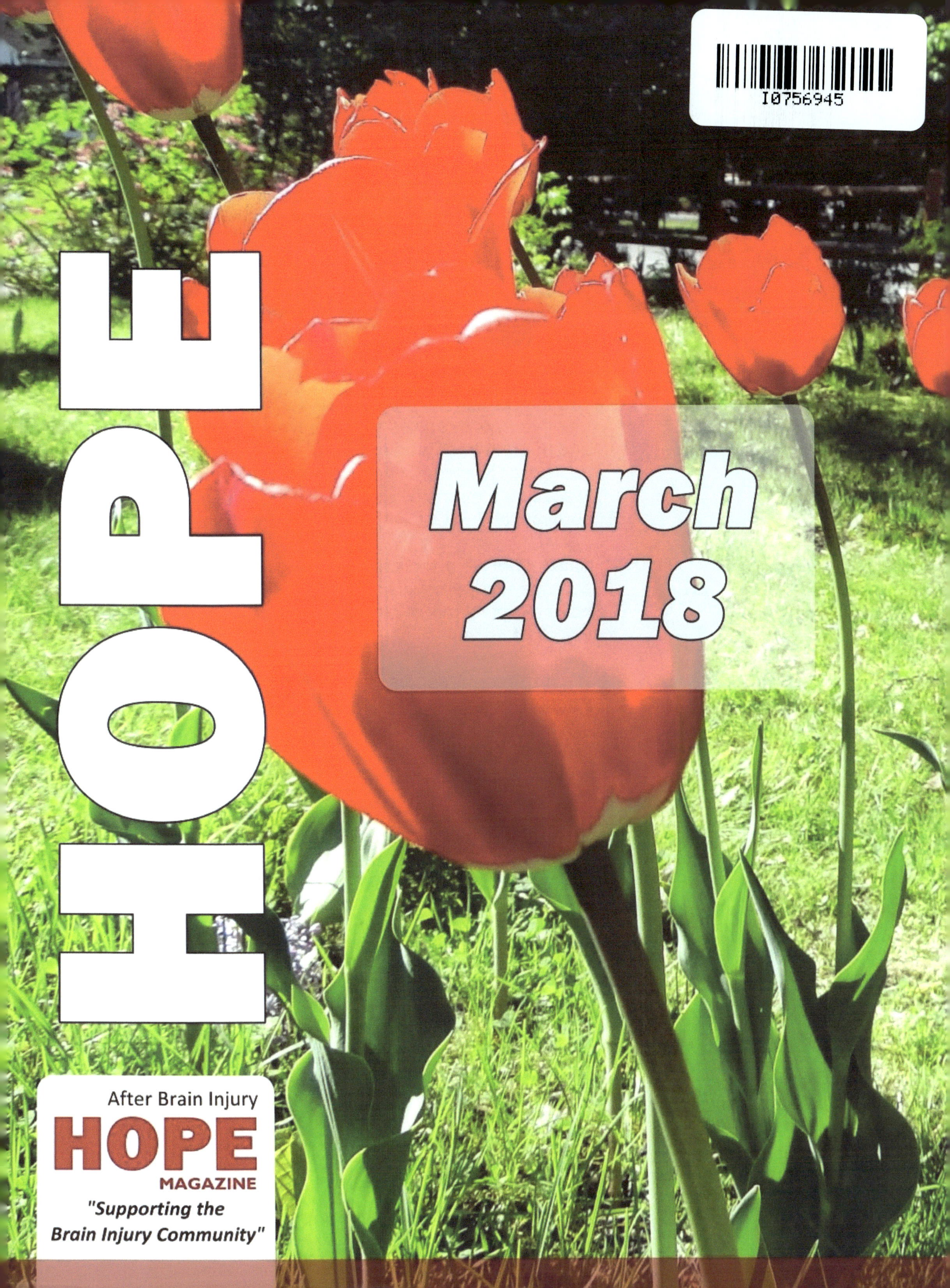

HOPE
March 2018
After Brain Injury
HOPE
MAGAZINE
"Supporting the
Brain Injury Community"

Welcome

HOPE MAGAZINE

Serving All Impacted by Brain Injury

March 2018

Publisher
David A. Grant

Editor
Sarah Grant

Contributing Writers
Haley Anderson
Michelle Bartlett
Gordon Brown
Sarah Kilch Gaffney
Adam Hapworth
Bob Milsap
Kellie Pokrifka
Lisa Yee
Connie Zanoni

*FREE subscriptions at
www.TBIHopeMagazine.com*

Welcome to the March 2018 issue of HOPE Magazine!

As most people within the brain injury community know, this is Brain Injury Awareness Month. This month offers a great opportunity to shine the spotlight on brain injury of all kinds.

Our March issue is very special for a couple of reasons. This month marks the three-year anniversary of HOPE Magazine and the one-year anniversary of our print version. In three short years, our readership has circled the globe, making HOPE Magazine the most widely read within the brain injury community.

This month we are pleased to bring you stories of hope, courage and perseverance against overwhelming odds. We have a perfect mix of past contributors as well as a few new voices of hope.

We also have a special section in this month's issue: *Young People and Brain injury.* The stories shared in this section show that hope can indeed be found, and lives rebuilt.

Peace,

David A. Grant
Publisher

Contents

"Nothing can be done without hope and confidence."
~Helen Keller

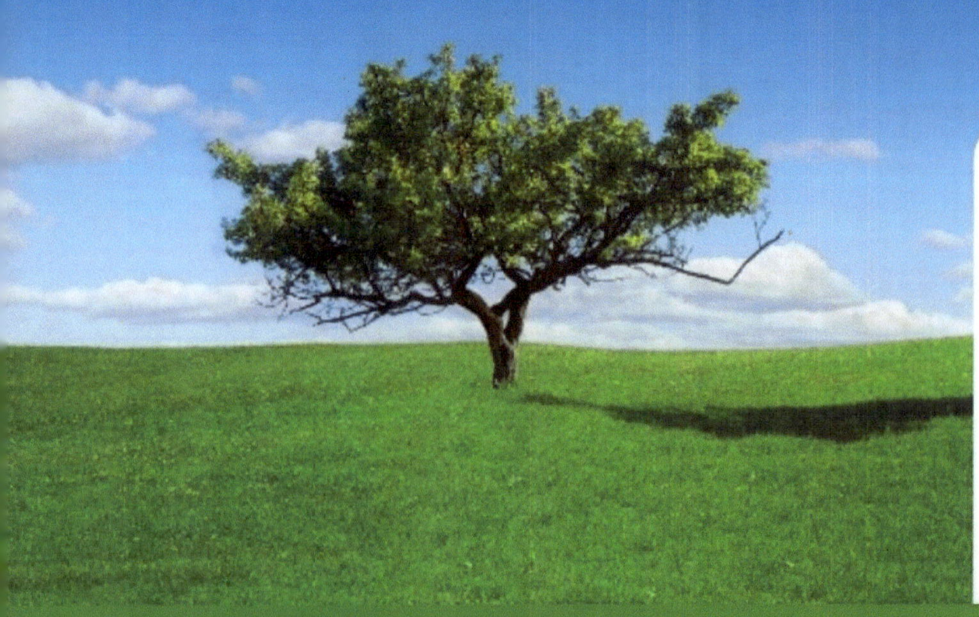

Our Mission

The Mission of the

HOPE After Brain Injury Network

is to Advocate, Educate, and Serve all

Affected by Brain Injury.

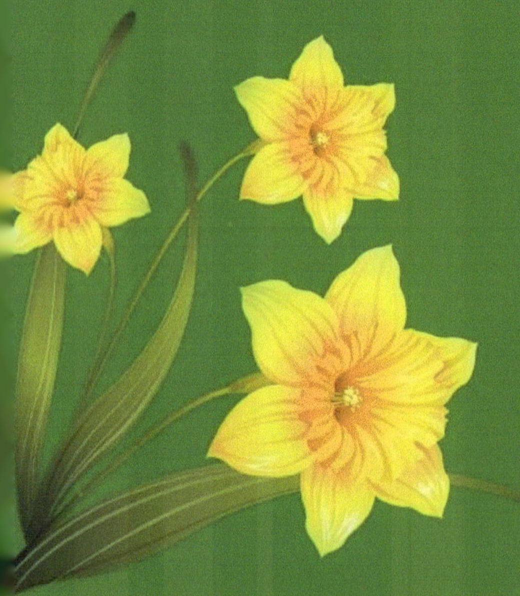

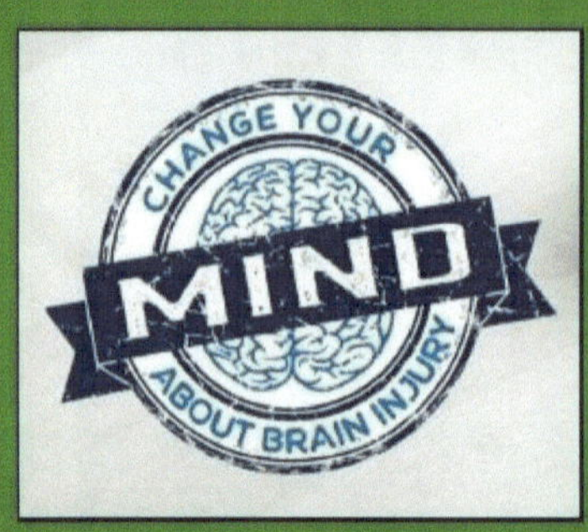

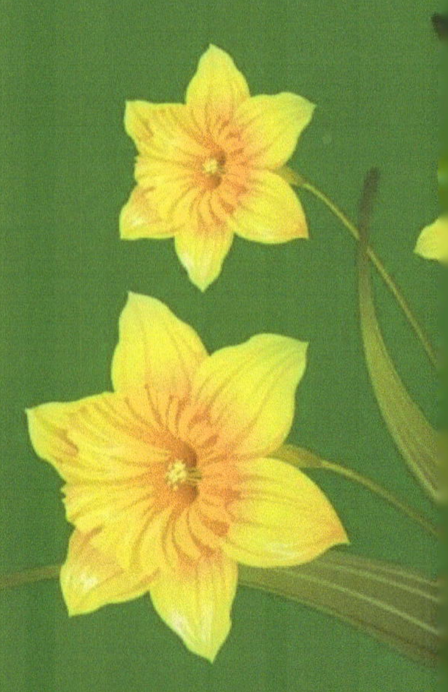

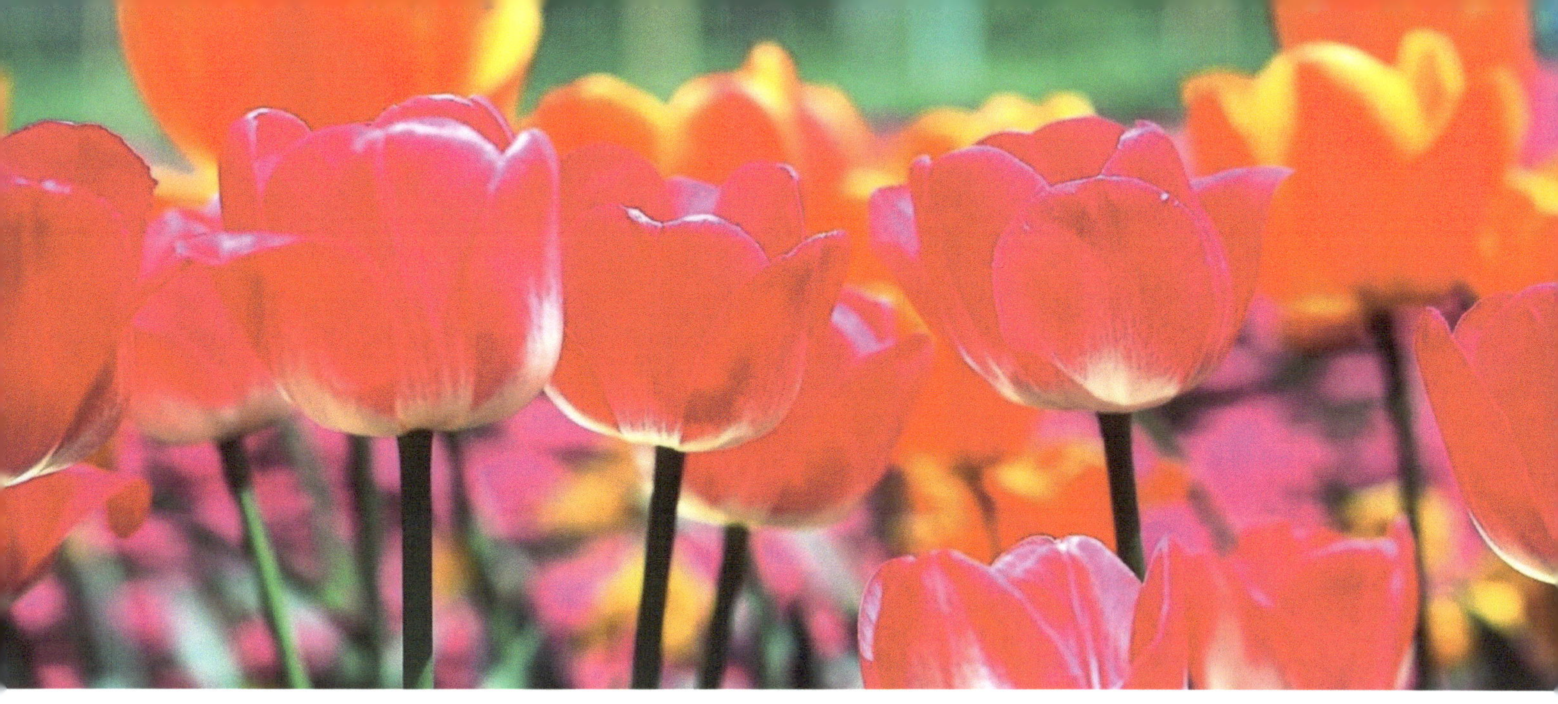

No Such Thing as Impossible

By Michelle Bartlett

March is a time of renewal, rebirth, and rejuvenation. After a long, cold winter full of ice and snow, spring is returning to North America. The snow is melting, and the temperatures are rising. The cold arctic air is now being replaced by a gentle spring breeze.

It is very fitting that March is Brain Injury Awareness Month. March is a very important month in my life also. On March 6th, I had my brain injury after open heart surgery and spent ten to twelve days in a coma before I slowly started to regain consciousness. I celebrate my re-birthday on March 17th, on St. Patrick's Day. Green was always my favourite color.

This year will be fourteen years since my brain injury. I am proud to say, I have come a long way in the last fourteen years. The medical professionals told my family that I was clinically brain dead with no hope of survival.

My family recalls more of my survival during the initial days of my recovery. I recall that they never left. Countless nights and days were spent at the hospital by my bedside. Countless meals they helped feed me. Countless tears were shed. I always saw them being strong, patient and loving with me. All of them were my strength, my protectors, and my rocks. I knew they were there when I needed them the most.

Slowly I began re-learning how to live again.

Learning how to live again is a long, slow process and not easy. It is not easy for the survivor, and especially hard for the family to watch the survivor struggle to adjust and accept this new normal.

I struggled with daily tasks and wanted to be the "normal Michelle" I thought I should be. Accepting the "new Michelle" was still years away.

I fought my "permanently disabled, never to return to work again" label. It felt like I had been written off, just to be put in a corner of society. My identity was my work. I enjoyed it. I enjoyed my independence. The first blow to my self-confidence was when I tried to go back to work a few times, only to fail. It took a few more years before I realized and accepted my new life. I was looking forward to getting married. In the blink of an eye everything changed.

When I first became aware of my surroundings and started to recognize people, places and things, it felt like a struggle just to live each day. I saw what was difficult for me, but I didn't understand why it was difficult.

I'm not proud to admit this now, but it took me many more years to realize how much my brain injury impacted my family and friends. I could not comprehend the impact it had on my family and friends. I had fallen into the trap that many survivors fall in: lack of insight.

I first had to become aware and accept the new Michelle.

I took baby steps. Some things I failed at, most I succeeded. My confidence grew leaps and bounds as I gradually regained my self-confidence and self-esteem. I grew up in a large, close-knit family. My Aunt and Sister-in-Law sent me emails to practice my writing skills. Mom and I were close and we did everything together. My Mother-in-Law and I were close and we spoke every day.

So many people did so many kind and generous things for both my family and myself. All of my family and friends were always there, gently nudging me along the way. If I forgot a word, they would wait and let me find it on my own.

We all got frustrated. There were many days that it seemed like there was no end, no peace, and no final chapter. Somehow we found it. My circle of people is much smaller than it was fourteen years ago. As much as I miss the friendships, love and support, it's okay - I understand. They needed to have a meaningful life too. Some people I miss more than I should.

Brain injuries are invisible injuries. To see me or talk to me on the street, you would never know I have had a brain injury. Most people do not know unless I tell them, but the compound effect on family and friends are astronomical and overwhelming. They are our unsung heroes and deserve more credit than they get.

I was lucky I had a good family and support system of friends. That made a huge difference in my recovery. Thank you to all my caregivers, friends and supporters – both past and present. I am living proof that with lots of work, patience, and support, there is no such thing as impossible.

Meet Michelle Bartlett

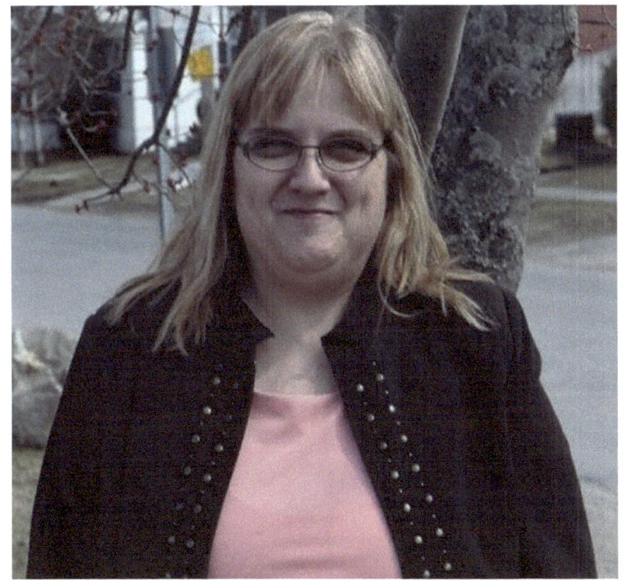

Michelle is a community advocate as well as a facilitator for brain injury survivors and their families and supporters. She suffered a severe anoxic brain injury in 2004 and has become very interested in brain injuries and psychology. She wants to learn and understand, and give back to the community that helped both her and her family during a very difficult time in their lives. She has come a long way from the early days being unable to care for herself and still has a long journey ahead of her. Now as an advocate for Brain Injury Canada, she feels strongly that she has a voice for the people that sometimes feel that their voices cannot be heard.

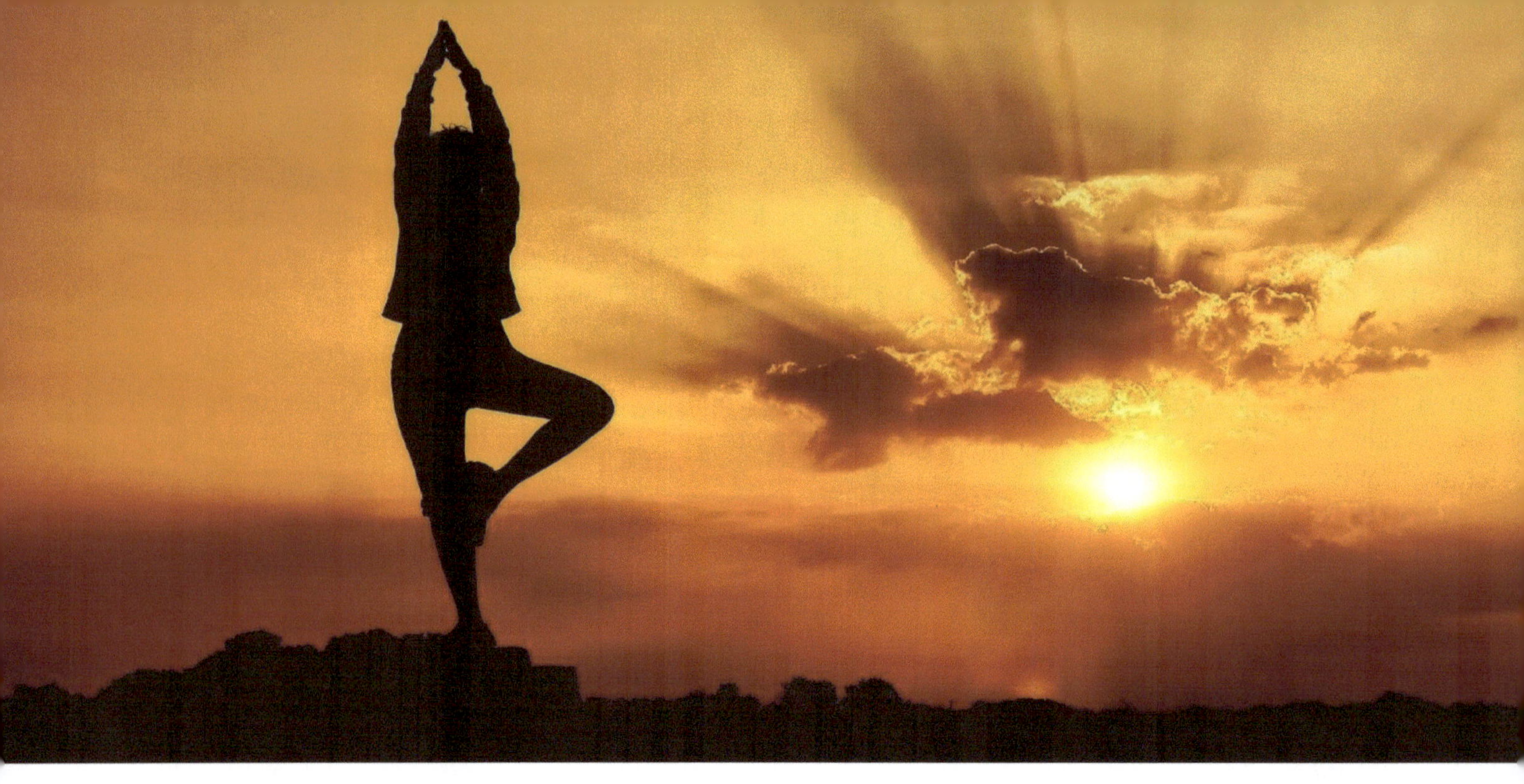

From Injury to Enlightenment
By Lisa Yee

I don't remember anything about the 2008 car crash we now call "The Accident." Only much later did my husband realize why a medic, calling for him to meet us at Loyola University Medical Center in Chicago as I was being loaded into a helicopter, urged him to hurry. It was to give him a chance to say goodbye.

When I awoke in the hospital a week later, with a broken body and a traumatic brain injury, no one knew if I'd ever be the same. After a month, I still couldn't retain short-term memories. I'd recognized my husband and daughter right away (but how had she gotten older?) No problem recalling Dad or my many siblings either, but I kept asking if Mom was still alive. She had died of cancer in 2007.

Such is the sometimes amusing, sometimes emotionally wrenching and always baffling world of the TBI patient. According to brainline.org, a TBI is *"a blow or jolt to the head or a penetrating head injury that disrupts the function of the brain."* Brain injuries affect 1.7 million people a year and cause 52,000 deaths in the United States alone.

> I kept asking if Mom was still alive. She had died of cancer in 2007.

In my case, the diagnosis was "moderate" TBI. Among other scary things I've found in trying to review the data my husband has summarized into a 3-inch-thick binder over the years, this diagnosis had to do with my rating on the Glasgow Coma Scale (not so good, apparently), my "initial decerebrate posture"

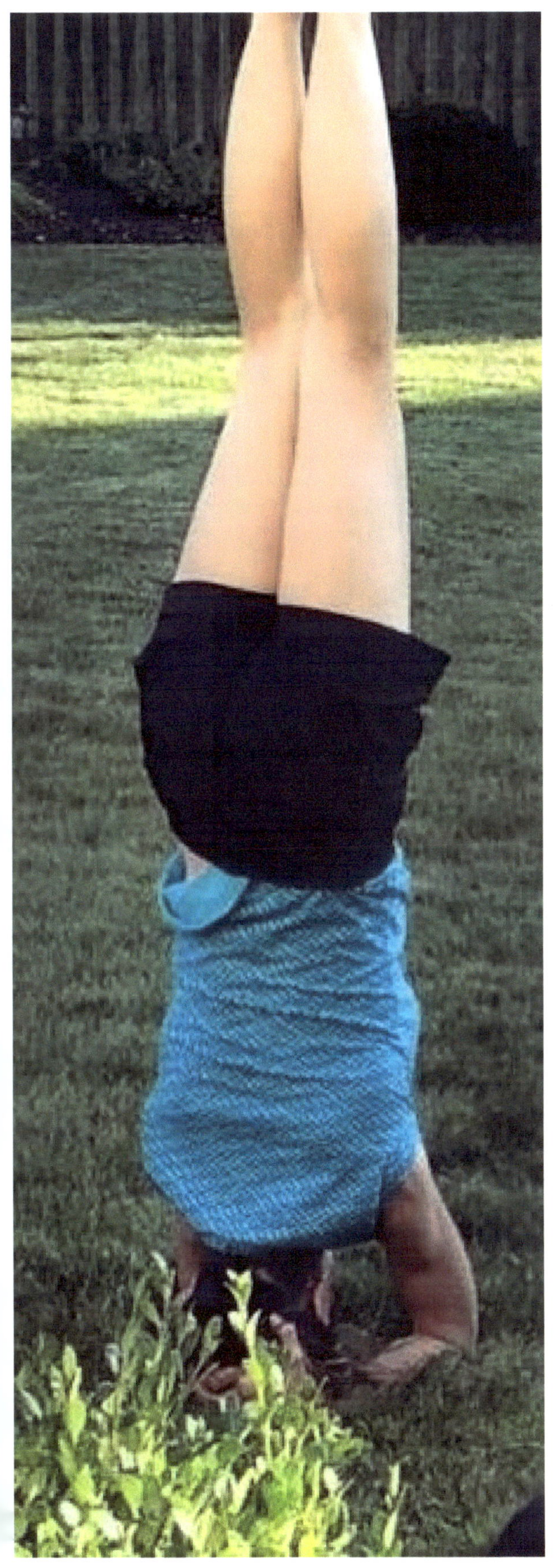

(a rigid body position with legs straight, toes down and neck arched) and seizures. I also read about my "months of physical and cognitive therapy" and my "residual neuro-cognitive problems," depression, hampered mobility and trouble with "activities of daily living." As much as I resisted it, we arranged for a home-care assistant.

Finally, I looked through my husband's transcription of my "seizure diary," a combination of my thoughts and his descriptions of my seizures, some of which he'd captured on video so the doctors could witness them. This trip down "no-memory lane" was my attempt to figure out the year I started yoga (was it 2011 or 2012? I'm not so good with numbers anymore), but I couldn't stop reading about my now-extremely rare episodes. This one, from March 2012, was from a night Ted was working late:

"I get ready for bed early, multitasking brushing my teeth on the john, when I hear my phone. Feel a seizure coming on and lean forward. Next thing I remember, Ted's home and he's coming to bed. It's hours later. I'd gotten myself cleaned up, into bed, lights out. (Discover a sore on outside of lip the next day, another inside— from my teeth. Also blood and toothpaste in my hair.)"

Today, as we approach our nine-year "Acci-versary," it's hard to identify with that version of myself, a newspaper editor forced to face a new reality. So much has changed — my physical recovery and return to fitness, new neurologists, the right medications, a deeper relationship with my husband … and yoga.

Ted (who's become so knowledgeable that people think he's a doctor) had urged me to try tai chi for its intense focus. I wanted something more athletic, so the instructor directed me to a yoga class taught by his wife, Lynda.

I now understand why Ted was drawn to focusing techniques like tai chi as a therapy for me.

In Dr. Norman Doige's 2007 bestseller, "The Brain That Changes Itself," the author discusses why people tend to become forgetful as they age. He explains that the nucleus basalis, a group of neurons in the brain, is designed to secrete acetylcholine, which helps form clear memories. Those neurons get neglected from a lack of mental stimulation, or from being "set in our ways."

"Anything that requires *highly focused attention* will help that system — new physical activities, challenging puzzles, new careers that require learning new skills," neuroscientist Michael Merzenich says in the book. He also touts the brain benefits of learning a new language in adulthood (Sanskrit, anyone?) and getting "sensory input from our feet."

I began attending classes three times a week, jogging the mile to the community center since I no longer drove. It felt good to work my muscles in new ways and to see myself in the big mirror holding (what I considered) perfect poses. But soon something inside me began to change. I'd catch a glimpse of my face in that mirror, and I'd be grinning, not grimacing. I'd see a classmate's pose and think, "You can do it!" instead of feeling self-conscious or competitive (my default modes). And after class, I'd feel calm.

These are not unusual effects of yoga and meditation, of "being in the present moment," I have learned.

Antoine Lutz, Ph.D., and Richard Davidson of the University of Wisconsin at Madison, have studied "Vipassana" or "insight" meditation for years. According to Psychology Today (Dec. 12, 2012), they found that the practice improved emotional regulation and stress control even when their test subjects were not meditating. When the researchers trained a different group in "compassion meditation" — having them focus on loved ones and then wish them "well-being and freedom from suffering" — this group showed evidence of increased empathy. In the brain, that was evidenced by more activation in the right amygdala in response to images of human suffering.

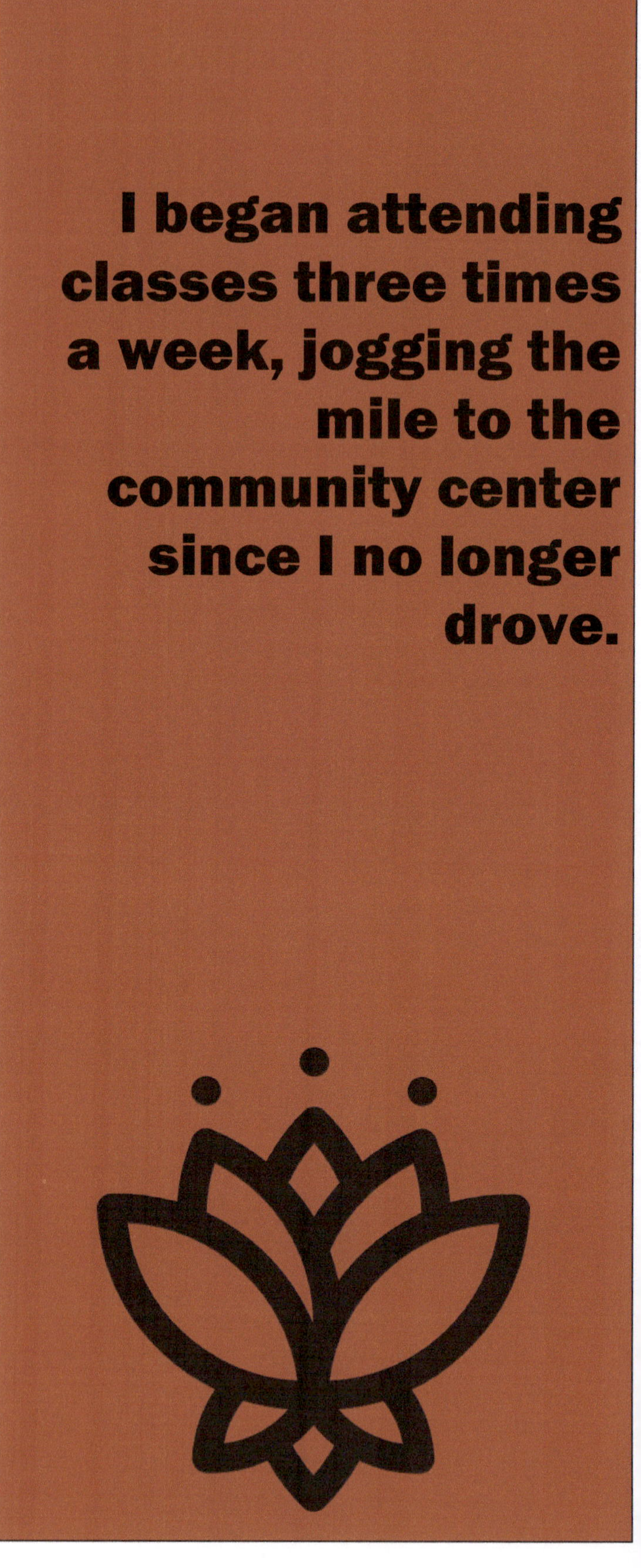

Interestingly, the compassion group also showed reduced rates of depression, as measured by psychological tests. "Davidson and Lutz's work suggests that through mindfulness training, people can develop skills that promote happiness and compassion," Psychology Today says. "People are not just stuck at their respective set points. We can take advantage of the brain's plasticity and train it to enhance these qualities."

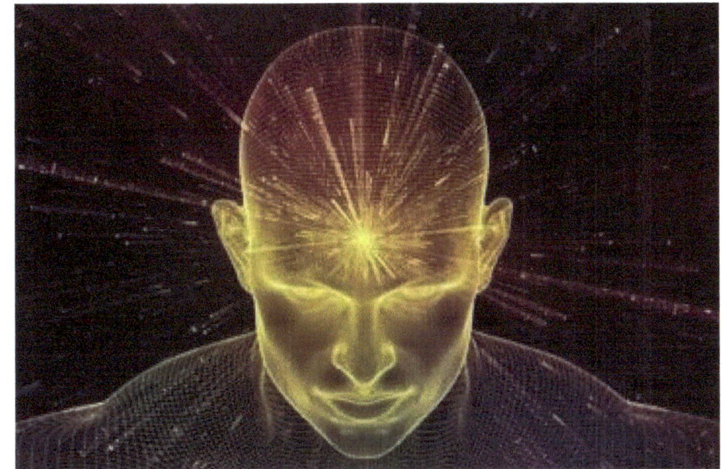

I remember hearing a lot about neuroplasticity, even in the early days, when I didn't quite know what Ted was talking about. What it means is the brain is capable of growing and changing over time, depending on how you use it. Doige explains it much better in "The Brain That Changes Itself:"

"Clearly, when we learn, we increase what we know, but we can also change the very structure of the brain itself and increase its capacity to learn. Unlike a computer, the brain is constantly adapting."

But the old "use-it-or-lose-it" principle is at work here as well. "Merzinich thinks our neglect of intensive learning as we age leads the systems in the brain that modulate, regulate and control plasticity to waste away," Doige says.

Hmm. At this point, I'm thinking I'd better back up and fill you in on the rest of my lingering… let's say, "peculiarities."

What people don't see (unless they're my husband) are the emotional fragility, the intense need for routine, and especially the mental fogginess when it's nearing time for my ten to twelve hours of nightly sleep.

There are a number of deficits in the brain's executive functioning that are *so* me:

- **Processing speed.** This is why, when new yoga cues are given, I often tilt my head quizzically and then just copy what my neighbor is doing.
- **Attention span.** Oh, look! My cat just woke up!
- **Sensory overload.** I don't wear the dark glasses just to look like Mrs. Cool. Also, big crowds, noise? I'm outta there.
- **Word finding.** That's gotten much better, but … who did you say you were again?
- **Disinhibition.** Uh-oh. My childlike lack of decorum ("I'll break into song at the grocery store if I want to!")
- **Multitasking.** Gah! Go, away, cat, I'm trying to write a thesis.
- **Follow-through.** Oh, I'll write that one later …
- **Sense of humor.** Ha! See above.

Numerous other studies have pointed to the benefits of yoga and meditation for TBI patients.

One study that I found especially interesting was the yoga program for soldiers returning from Afghanistan and Iraq at Eisenhower Army Medical Center in Fort Gordon, Georgia. Dr. John Rigg, director of the TBI Clinic at the base, describes on NPR's *All Things Considered*, how a blast in combat can affect a soldier.

"What happens is that primitive animal instinct, which is located in the subcortical brain, becomes hyper-aroused. … The subcortical brain doesn't understand geography and stays hyper-aroused. Their muscles are tightened up."

But after a short time in yoga, he says, participants report better sleep, relaxed muscles and a better outlook. "It's an enlightening factor, even for people who don't continue in yoga, to see that they can use breath and physical movement to actually change the way they feel."

In other brain-positive research, a 2013 study at Beth Israel Deaconess Medical Center in Boston compared MRI scans of cognitively impaired people after an eight-week program of yoga, meditation and mindfulness with those of similar patients who had gotten standard care. According to the April-May 2015 edition of Neurology Now, the program group showed better connectivity in the hippocampus, which is related to learning and memory. (Score! The hippocampus is where most of my damage is!)

> **Other benefits, as measured by physical assessments and interviews, were confidence, lower-extremity strength and endurance.**

And then there's this, from the June 2015 edition of the medical journal Disability and Rehabilitation: An eight-week mixed-methods case study in which yoga teachers worked individually with TBI patients showed a 36 percent improvement in balance (a biggie for me; I still struggle with those types of poses). Other benefits, as measured by physical assessments and interviews, were confidence, lower-extremity strength and endurance. Said one patient: "I mean, it's rocked my world. It's changed my life—I mean, all the different aspects. I mean, physically, emotionally, mentally—it's given me, you know, my life back."

Physically, emotionally, mentally. … I know, right? But for me there's more.

It's hard to describe, but I feel a new sense of connectedness now. Things happen because they're supposed to happen; everything works out. If The Accident made me who I am today, I'm glad. I like myself better now. I think this awareness came several years later, when I was no longer in "survival" mode, going from seizure to seizure, so maybe my brain had a chance to heal somewhat.

The feeling grew when I started yoga — and *exploded* when I learned to meditate. In fact, shortly after a three-day meditation seminar at Prairie by visiting teacher Nicolai Bachman — that, honestly, did not hold my interest — I became aware of a strange phenomenon. When I closed my eyes, I could "see" what looked like an open eye at about the bridge of my nose. Being an idiot, I mentioned this to a classmate, figuring it was some bizarre "neurological thingy" from my old TBI. She said something like, "Whoa, that's really advanced." So I did some reading (in my own Teacher Training Manual, for gosh sakes) and concluded that I was seeing that famed "Third Eye" that lets you "see from a deeper place" and "trust your own intuition."

Whoa, indeed. Or, maybe I'm just nuts.

But my shrink assures me I'm not. "Your participation in yoga helped you to shift to a level of being more peaceful inside," says psychologist Joseph Keegan of Naperville, with whom I've worked for I-forget-how-many years now. "Prior to that, you were at more of a frenetic pace—anxious, pensive. Yoga provided you with a sense of equanimity and altered your sense of interconnection with the world."

He says yoga "opened up a door to a sense of spirituality" and even points out that my habit of picking up litter and recycling as I walk home "reflects that you feel you have a place in the universe."

I guess the point of all this is that yoga and meditation — plus music, nature, friends, family (especially a devoted, selfless spouse) and faith — are the keys to coping with brain injury.

Meet Lisa Yee

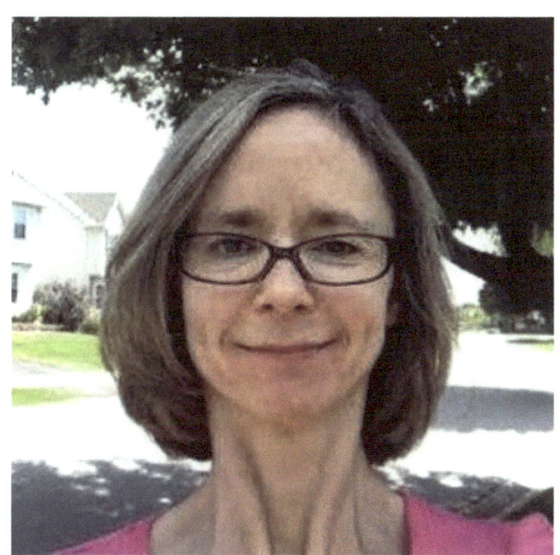

Lisa Yee of suburban Chicago suffered a traumatic brain injury/epilepsy in a 2008 car accident. Before her injury, she had been a newspaper editor for two decades after graduating from the Indiana University School of Journalism. It was there she met her husband, Ted. They have a daughter, Megan, of Chicago.

Post TBI, Lisa became certified as a yoga instructor and now volunteers teaching yoga at a women's shelter and a veterans center.

INTRODUCING THE NEW
dish FLEX PACK
Create Your Own TV Package

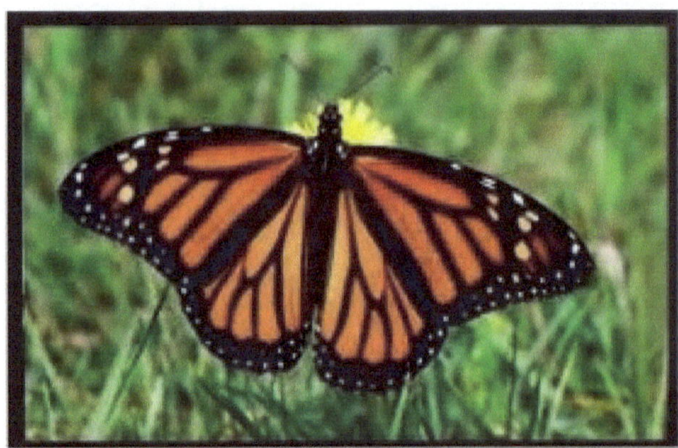

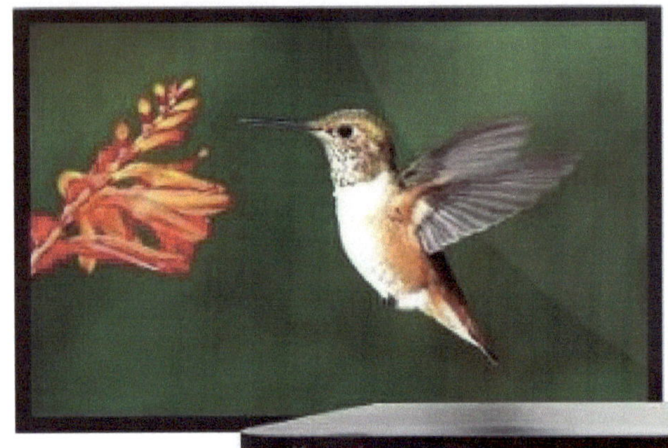

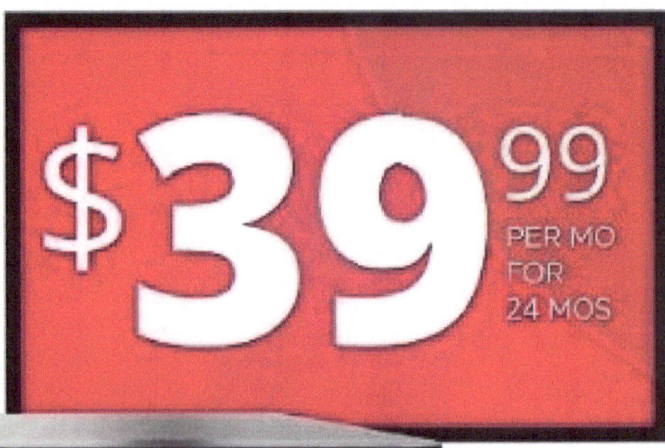

Free Streaming

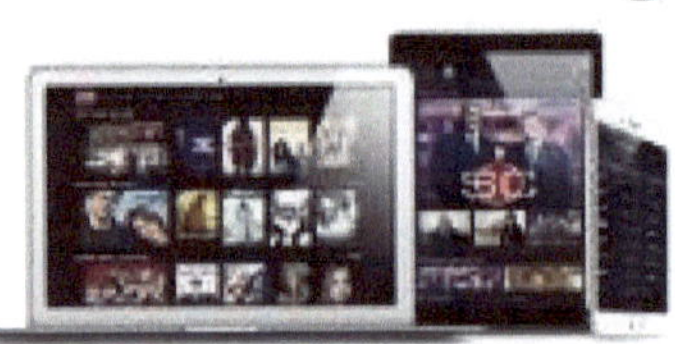
on all of your devices

+

Free Installation

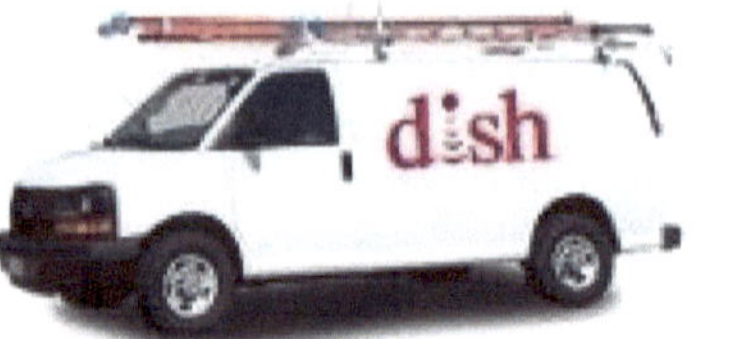

+

Add Internet

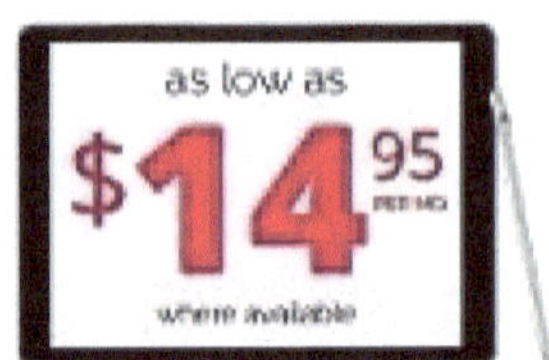

Call 1-800-391-1328

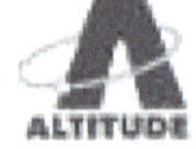

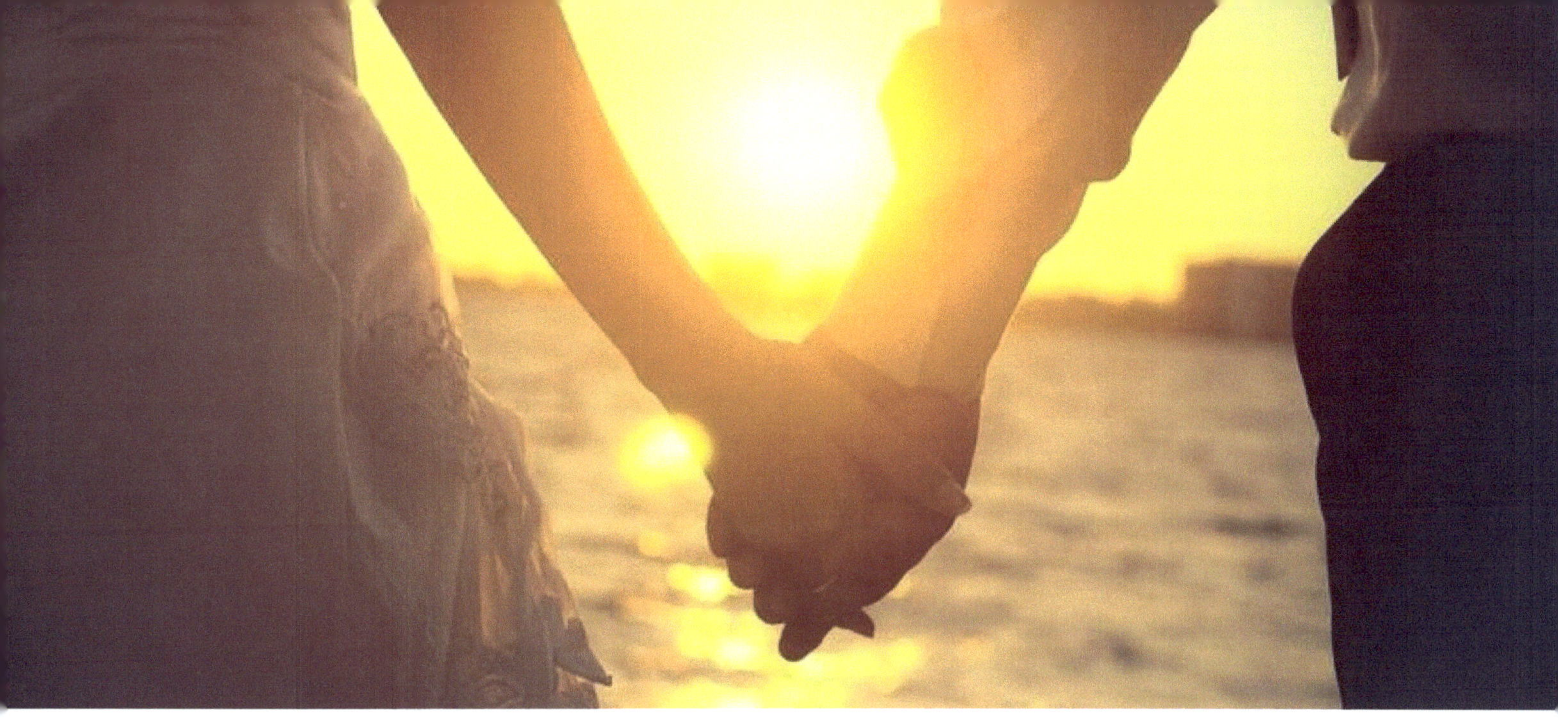

My Wife, My Inspiration
By Bob Milsap

The five-year anniversary of my wife Shelly's traumatic brain injury passed last week. Her life, and our entire family's life, was forever changed in a split second on that cold day in January of 2013. We had a freak accident happen within our home. A homemade bottle of ginger ale was taken from the refrigerator to the kitchen sink to be poured out. Shelly was busy and did not pour it out right away. As it sat on the counter for a few days, it went from cold to warm, and it slowly fermented. As it fermented, it turned into a bomb. The bomb happened to detonate at the exact instance that Shelly walked past it in the kitchen. The force of the blast through the tiny opening of the 2-liter bottle knocked Shelly unconscious to the ground. We estimate that she regained consciousness about twenty minutes later. She was bloody, her face was swollen and there was ginger ale splattered all over the kitchen.

Dazed, she called me immediately. I was at work, running a natural foods store in Jackson Hole, Wyoming. It took me a bit to understand what had happened. She sent me a picture of her face. I was horrified at the sight of her swollen, bloody, black and blue face. We lived in tiny and remote Victor, Idaho. I called neighbors to see if anyone was home to take her to the doctor.

> "I look back now and realize how foolish I was in not calling an ambulance."

Everyone I talked to had already made the commute to Jackson Hole for the day. I look back now and realize how foolish I was in not calling an ambulance. Nonetheless, Shelly got herself to the car, which was covered in ice. It was zero degrees outside.

Between scraping the windshield and running the defroster for several minutes, she was able to see out of a tiny corner of the windshield and she drove the mile to the Victor's lone health clinic.

The nurse and doctor that immediately saw Shelly were appalled at the sight of her face. They immediately thought she had been a victim of domestic violence. Shelly was able to explain what had happened and the doctor quickly called me. I was on my way to cross the mountainous Teton Pass on the thirty-minute drive home to Idaho. The doctor was extremely concerned about Shelly's eye and nose and thought that both her nose and eye socket were broken. She told me the nurse would be driving her to the small hospital in the town of Driggs, which was ten miles north of Victor.

I navigated the ice-packed roads to meet Shelly at the hospital. I could not believe how black, blue and swollen Shelly's face was. The result of the CT scan came quickly. The hospital doctor explained that her nose was broken, but her eye socket was not. She told us how fortunate she was that this was the only extent to Shelly's injuries.

We went home very confused as to how this kind of accident could happen, but also feeling lucky that this was the extent of it. As we entered the kitchen at home, we saw sticky ginger ale everywhere. I also saw the 2-liter soda bottle lying on the ground, intact. The bottle cap was in the dining room. I cleaned up, Shelly rested, and we counted our blessings.

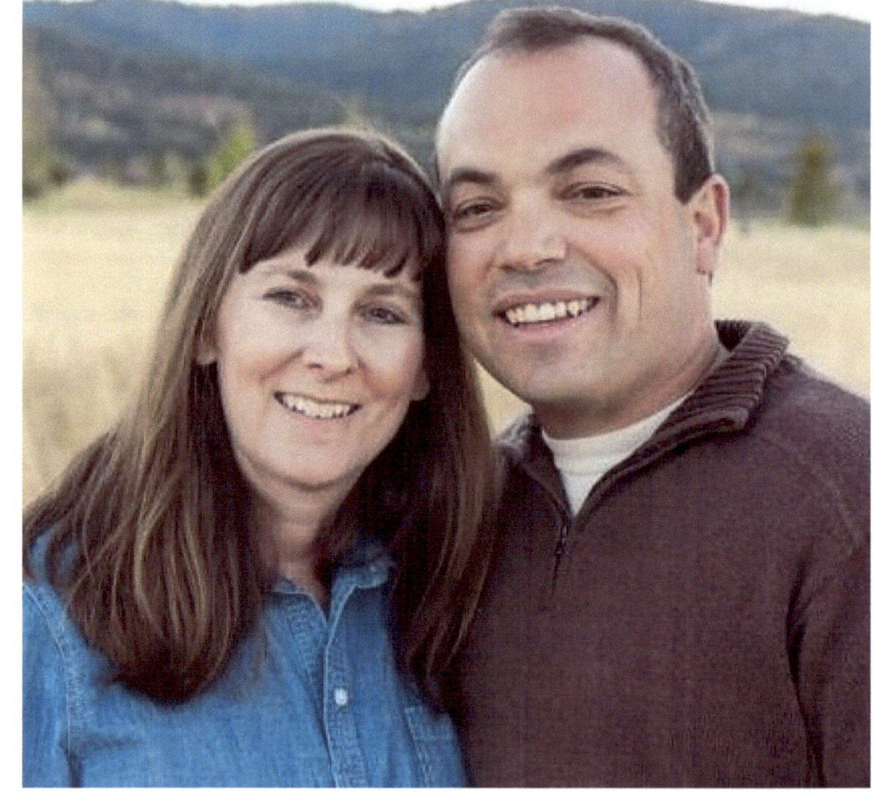

The next day Shelly went back to work. She recently started a baking business that had really taken off. She shrugged off her injuries and dug into her many baking orders at the nearby commercial kitchen that she rented space in. As the days passed, her nose and face hurt, but she was healing up and life was getting back to normal.

Fifteen days after the accident, Shelly called me at work to ask me to bring food home for dinner. She started to talk, but couldn't get the words out. Panic stricken, I quickly left work and drove home. I called the doctor and told her what had happened. She told me that we needed to see a neurologist right away. The neurologist only visited our remote valley twice a month, but explained that he would be there tomorrow and for us to come in. As I rushed into our house, I was greeted by Shelly sitting in the living room. She struggled to talk and could barely walk. I was numb with shock.

That next day, we visited the neurologist. He told me that Shelly was much like a soldier that was hit by a bomb at war. She had a traumatic brain injury and she would not be getting better. This was our "new normal," and I needed to adjust to it. He said this all in such a matter-of-fact way. This gentleman certainly lacked bedside manner! At one point he asked Shelly why she talked in such an "infantile" way.

From that day forward the true journey began. I quickly realized that there must be better care than this rude, insensitive doctor. Walking and talking had become so difficult, she was having to learn how to do it again. Parts of both her short and long-term memory were gone. I was working for someone who turned out to be a non-compassionate jerk, and who did not like that I needed to cut my workload from 70+ hours per week to 55 or so. We had no family nearby. We moved to the Tetons less than two years earlier, so Shelly had not made close friends yet. We were isolated, alone, and facing bigger hurdles than anyone could imagine. We had two children that quickly stepped up and helped however they could. Dylan was 17, and Taylor was 12.

The closest large city to us was Salt Lake City, Utah. It was five hours away. I made an appointment at the University Of Utah's Neurology Department. Shelly was furious with me and did not want to go. She did not realize how severe her situation was and how she desperately needed help. In Utah, I learned that we were extremely fortunate that Shelly did not lose her life that January day.

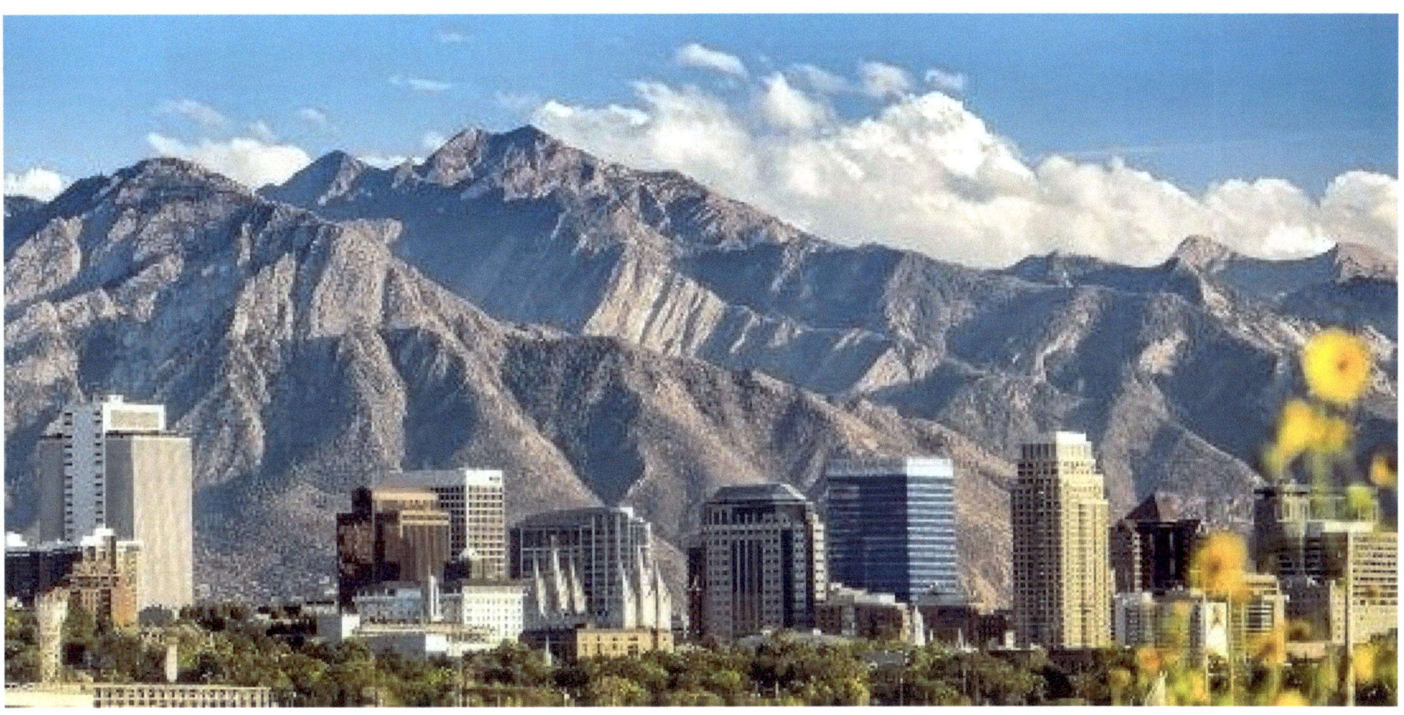

I was falling apart. I would cry uncontrollably as I drove to and from work. I was not a stranger to tragedy. My fiancée had been killed over twenty years earlier, and now I was driving down the road crying and saying, "why me again," and "why Shelly?" But, as I walked through the door at work or at home, I tried to appear to have it all together.

I had never considered Shelly a very patient person but, I was becoming amazed by how patient Shelly had become with herself and her situation. I was feeling sorry for her and for myself, but she would have none of that. She started working each and every day toward improvement. Baby steps were made. Fairly quickly we discovered that western medicine does not know how to really handle traumatic brain injury: the answer seemed to be to over medicate every symptom. Medical professionals had limited answers on how to truly treat the root of the problem.

We also learned that Shelly had what was called an "invisible injury." Her face healed up nicely and she looked great! People cannot understand how severely injured a person can actually be when they look great. Friends and family started to think she must be fine, since she looks so good. That was hard, because we needed so much help, but people didn't understand that at all.

We eased away from "Western medicine," more and more. There were a couple of local "alternative" medical providers that started to do wonders for Shelly. One provider worked on manipulating her central nervous system in a way that was re-wiring her brain cells. The other did amazing work with acupuncture and acupressure. We traveled to Arizona to learn "Neuro-feedback" treatment that we could do from home.

We would constantly experience small milestones. These were milestones such as driving to the corner to pick up Taylor at the bus stop, cooking a simple meal, or walking to the mailbox down the street. Shelly kept working so hard and was so aware of each improvement she had made. The milestones she achieved gradually became bigger and bigger. We had become very close as a family. Dylan, Taylor, and I were the only people that truly knew what a courageous battle Shelly was fighting. On the rare occasion that we would see friends or family, they would only get a small glimpse of her struggle. It was hard for them to truly understand the magnitude of the battle.

A little over a year-and-a-half ago we moved back to Arizona. I feel like this has been the single best thing for her. Friends, sunshine, and familiar surroundings have been amazing for her.

So many areas of her injury have improved. The post traumatic migraine headaches occur far less often. In my estimation, her motor skills are now 80% of what they were prior to her accident. Some of the areas greatly impacted include her mapping skills; she struggles with any type of multi-tasking. Simple math has become difficult. Areas of both her short and long-term memory are still affected. She spends hours each day doing brain exercises that help her continue to make improvements.

Post-Traumatic Stress Disorder (PTSD) is the biggest repercussion of her injury. The PTSD is still very severe. Her brain remains in constant panic mode. Noises, commotion, sudden and abrupt changes all create complete havoc in her brain. I have become extremely aware of our surroundings at all times. I try to quickly make appropriate adjustments when necessary. She is able to go to Taylor's varsity basketball and football games, but with earplugs and sitting away from the band and the majority of the crowd. She is able to drive the surface streets in our far western Phoenix suburbs and for a few miles on the freeway when traffic is light. But she certainly cannot drive across town on the interstate. The two worst nights of the year for her are the 4th of July and New Year's Eve, as the fireworks put her in uncontrollable tears and fear. There are so many examples of things that trigger her PTSD. To see her so quickly in

These were milestones such as driving to the corner to pick up Taylor at the bus stop, cooking a simple meal, or walking to the mailbox down the street.

such fear is both helpless and heartbreaking to me. My biggest goal for us is to find the proper treatment to help combat this PTSD "flooding."

I am Shelly's caregiver. There are many things that she can no longer do for herself. But being around her every day, I can't properly express how inspiring she is to me in her courageous daily battle. She deals with the ramifications of her brain injury and PTSD with such positivity and grace. I am in awe of her strength and optimism.

Shelly is truly my hero.

Meet Bob & Shelly Milsap

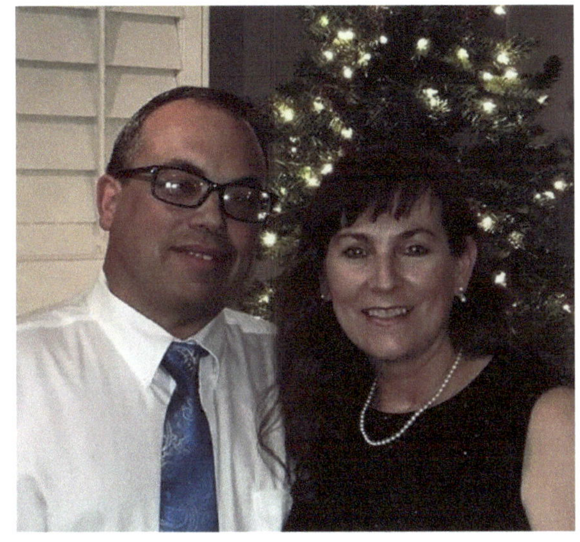

Five years ago my wife Shelly was involved in a freak accident that has forever changed her life. She suffered a traumatic brain injury that left her having to relearn to walk and talk again. She is saddled with severe PTSD, as her brain is in constant panic mode. I am Shelly's caregiver. There are many things that she can no longer do for herself. But being around her every day, I can't properly express how inspiring she is to me in her courageous daily battle. She deals with the ramifications of her brain injury and PTSD with such positivity and grace. I am in awe of her strength and optimism. I am sharing our story in hopes that it can help others in their journey.

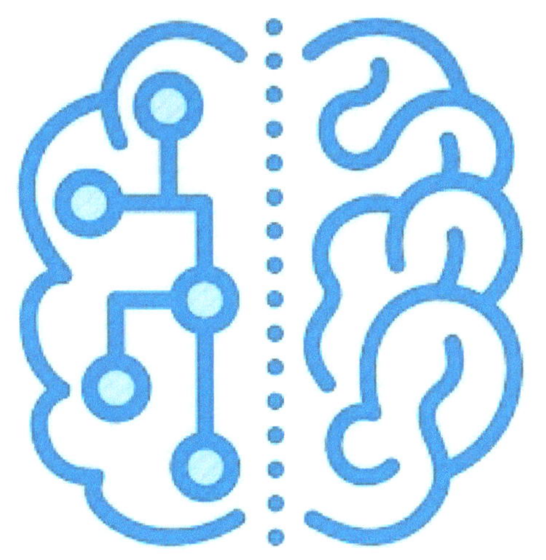

Neuroplasticity

The ability of the brain to form and reorganize synaptic connections, especially in response to learning or experience or following injury.

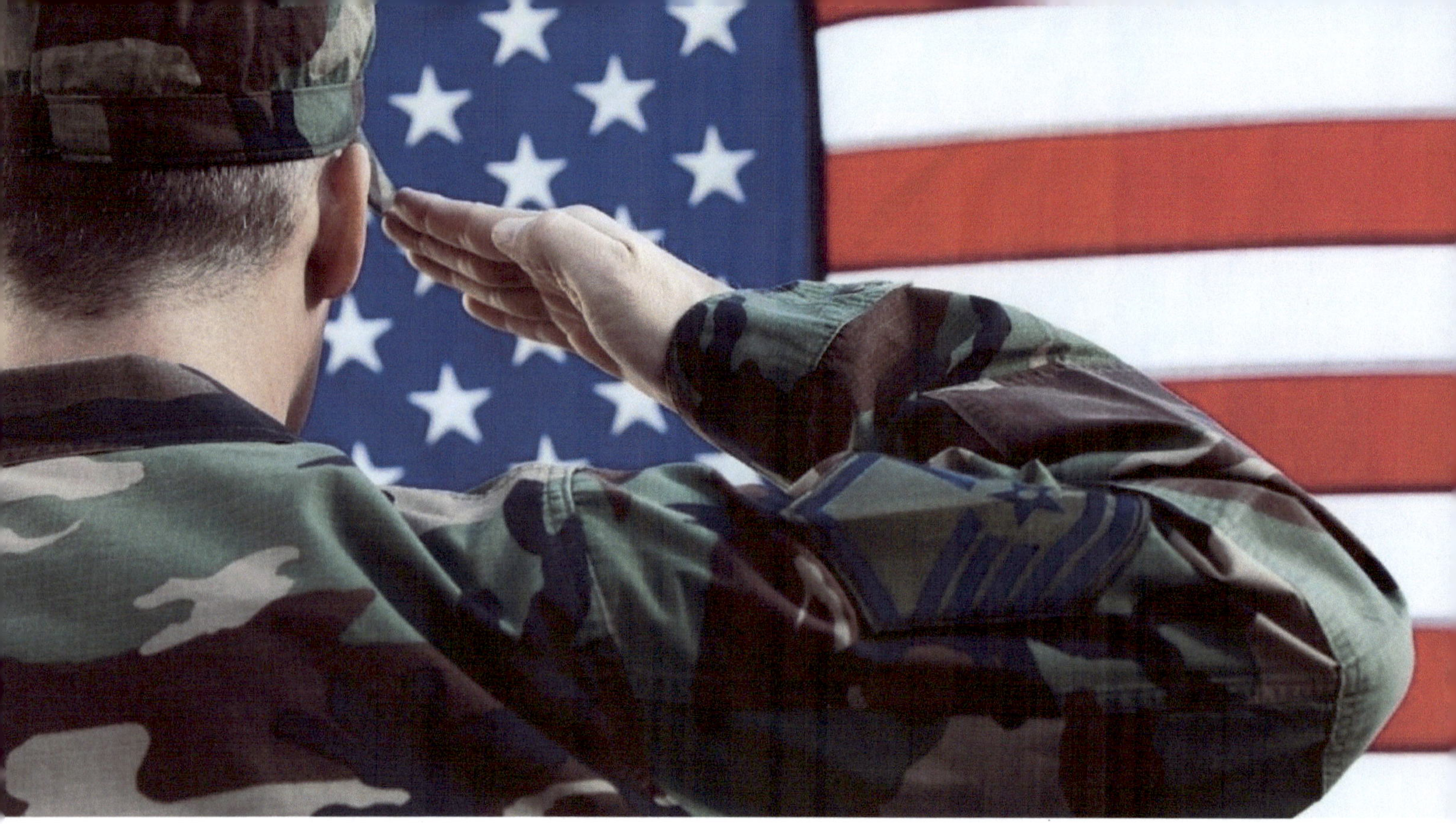

The Team Veteran Foundation

By Gordon Brown

I am the founder of Team Veteran Foundation and I am a survivor of a near fatal Traumatic Brain Injury (TBI). After a severe blow to the right side of my head I began bleeding on the brain. The bleeding continued for almost two months. I had a venous subdural hematoma and an MRI performed on 11/5/2002 showed predominantly white areas, indicating pools of blood.

I underwent emergency brain surgery that day. After surgery, I suffered two grand mal seizures and had a near death experience (NDE). I was placed on a daily dosage of 650mg of Dilantin and 750mg of Depakote to prevent future seizures. For three-and-one-half years, I took my medications and thought about suicide almost daily. After fighting the medication-induced suicidal thoughts, and a serious suicide attempt incident, I demanded to be taken off the Dilantin/Depakote cocktail. I was seconds away from being a statistic and being 1 of the 22-30 Veterans who die by suicide daily.

Living with the aftermath of a Traumatic Brain Injury (TBI) was a very frustrating and confusing process. I had trouble with speech, reading, long and short term memory, word searches, balance, sleep, and anger just to name a few. Talking with people I didn't know was extremely difficult, and that started a journey to find something to help with a more deliberate recovery.

I researched many different possible therapies and used cognitive rehabilitation therapy to help in relearning to read. I found that when I read, my eyes would stop tracking after about two sentences and I had 0% comprehension. I used audio books and the same version of the written book to force my eyes to track again. Two months later I was reading again.

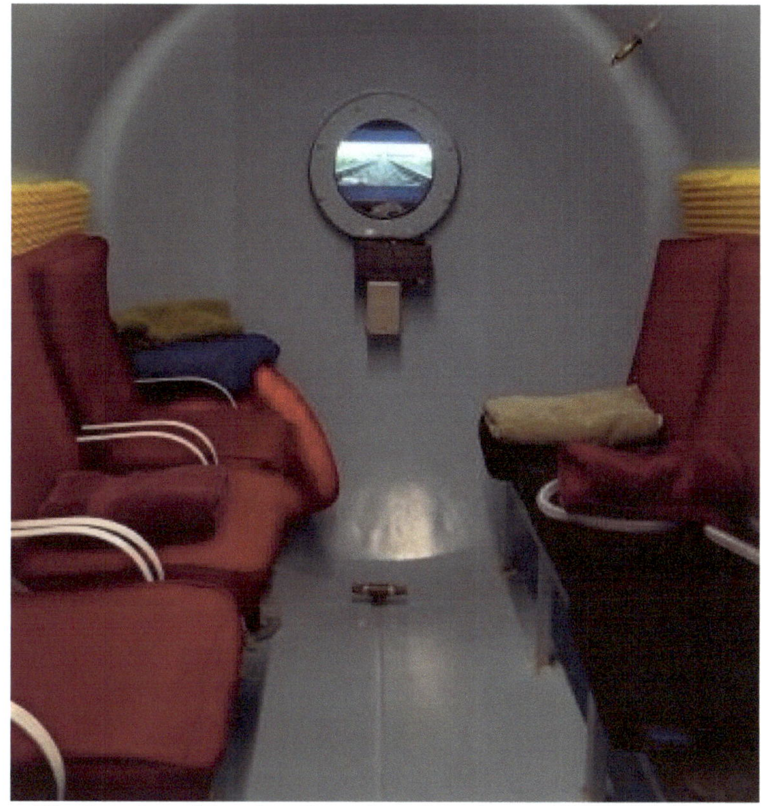
The interior of the chamber where I made my 40 HBOT dives.

My search took me down many paths, eventually leading me to a therapy called Hyperbaric Oxygen Therapy or HBOT. I became almost obsessed with learning all I could about HBOT and the potential to treat my physical brain injury. I started sponsoring Veterans who also suffered a TBI and was very excited to one day complete the forty one-hour "dives" which is the recommended HBOT protocol for a TBI. A "dive" is what the HBOT treatment is called because the chambers are used to treat SCUBA divers that are suffering from decompression sickness (DCS) also known as the "Bends."

I was contacted by someone in the HBOT field, who told me they had heard about what I was doing and offered to sponsor my forty dives. On September 21, 2015, I started the recommended forty one-hour dives in a multi-place Hyperbaric Oxygen Therapy chamber and finished the fortieth dive on November 13 of that year. The TBI negatively impacted my cognition and the HBOT dives returned my cognition to normal or better. If you believe that Veterans deserve a non-drug alternative therapy to treat their physical brain injuries, HBOT therapy is highly beneficial.

The incredibly positive changes I witness during my dives is why I am driven to create Team Veteran Foundation Wellness Clinics. These clinics will help bring a permanent end to the 22-30 daily Veteran suicides, which have become an epidemic. A suicide is like no other death for the family, the wound never heals. By empowering Veterans and their families suffering from the life threatening medical conditions of TBI and PTS with resources, support and services, we will make a difference. One of the cornerstone services of the Team Veteran Foundation Wellness Clinics is the Hyperbaric Oxygen Therapy (HBOT) chambers for the treatment of the physical brain injuries suffered during a Traumatic Brain Injury (TBI). As a Blue Water Navy Vietnam Veteran I was exposed to Agent Orange during my time in the Gulf of Tonkin, Vietnam and during my dives, I discovered HBOT aids in detoxing heavy metals and chemicals. It is my hope that sharing my story will help others on their own journey of recovery.

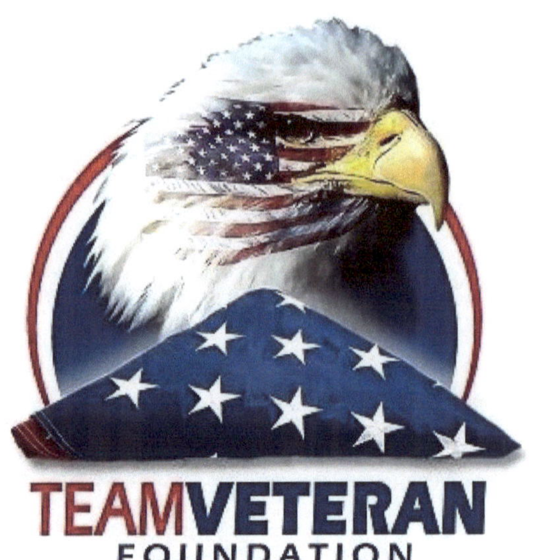

About Team Veteran Foundation, Inc.

Team Veteran Foundation, Inc., a 501(c)(3) is creating and aligning with wellness clinics that will be open seven days a week including holidays, utilizing Integrative Medicine therapies focusing on Hyperbaric Oxygen Therapy (HBOT) chambers to treat Traumatic Brain Injury (TBI) and Post-Traumatic Stress (PTS). We have a Veteran suicide epidemic with 22-30 Veterans dying daily from suicide. A suicide is like no other death for the family, the wound never heals. We are looking for those Patriots that can make charitable donations and realize they have already received their Return on Investment. That ROI is called Freedom. We need your help with this mission to #StopTheClock. Please visit www.tvfaz.org for more information.

Meet Gordon Brown

Gordon Brown is the founder of the nonprofit Team Veteran Foundation, Inc. and Team Veteran LLC, He served in the United States Navy during the Vietnam War 1972-1980, serving aboard the aircraft carriers USS Oriskany CVA/CV-34 and USS Ranger CV-61. He also served in Guam in the mid 1970's and worked with several government agencies to investigate and stop a major drug smuggling operation that was moving heroin from Thailand through the island of Guam, bound for the Continental US aboard Pan Am Airways.

Gordon transferred to the Naval Drug Rehabilitation Center (NDRC) at NAS Miramar, where he was promoted to Petty Officer, First Class. MM1 Brown was a Senior Counselor, Suicide Prevention Officer, Military Liaison Officer for Narcotics Anonymous, and initiated the therapy program that eventually became the standard core-therapy for the entire Naval Drug Rehabilitation programs worldwide. He proudly served in the United States Merchant Marines as an Engineering Officer from 1981-1993 and left the USNR as a LCDR. He is a service-connected disabled veteran and also experienced a near fatal Traumatic Brain Injury (TBI) in civilian life. This affords him a unique perspective on the challenges that face our Veterans and their families.

CELEBRATING

THREE YEARS OF HOPE

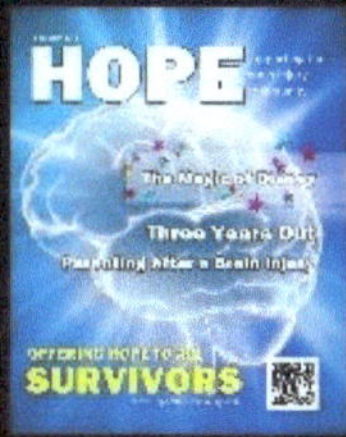
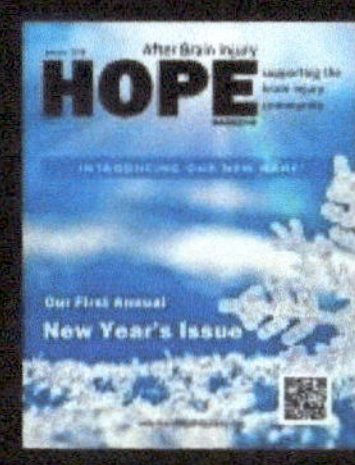
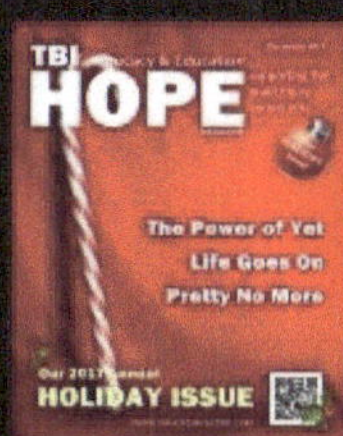
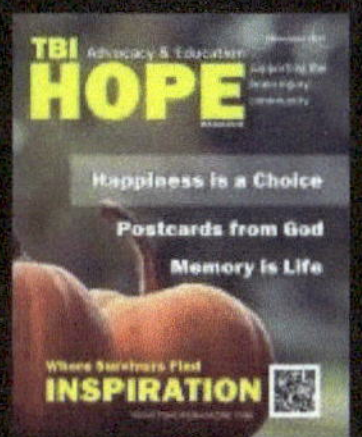
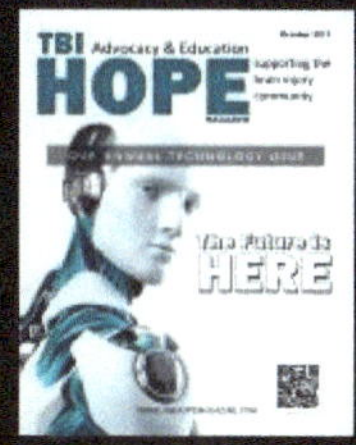
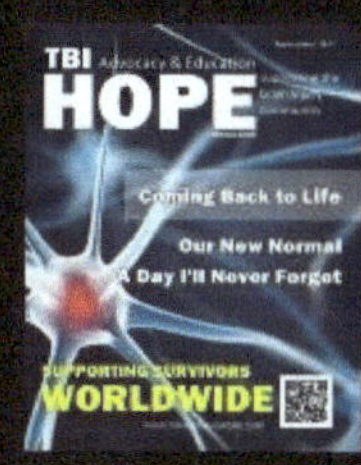
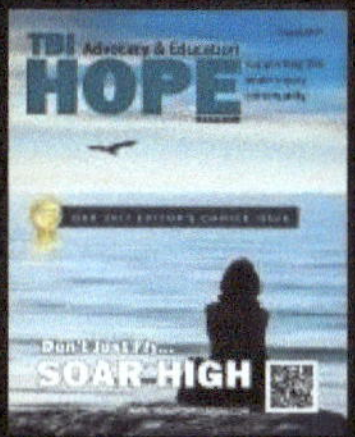
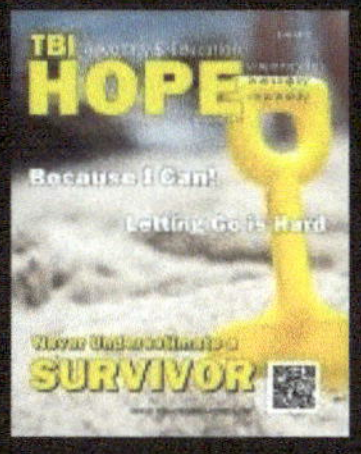
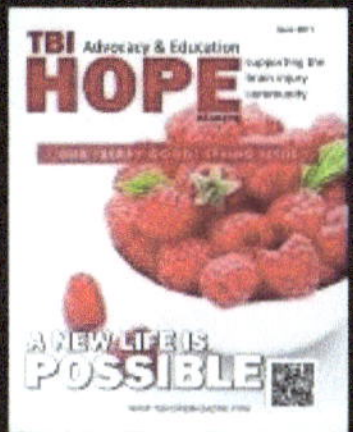
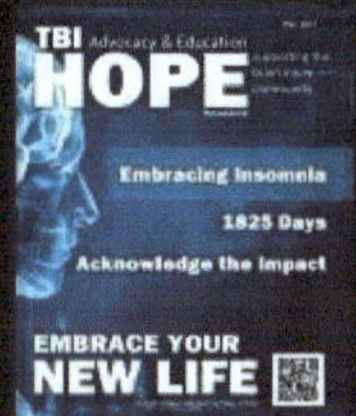
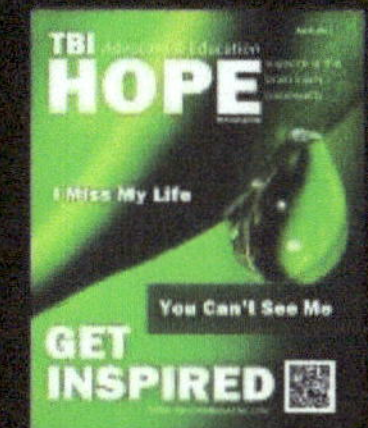
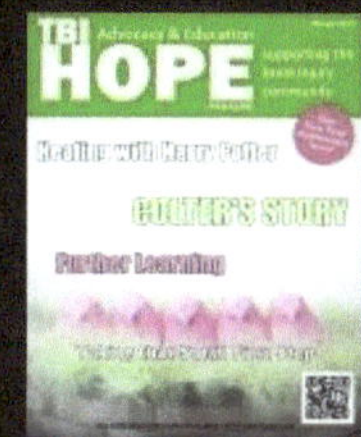
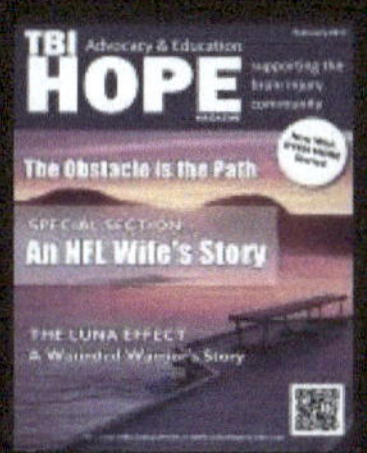
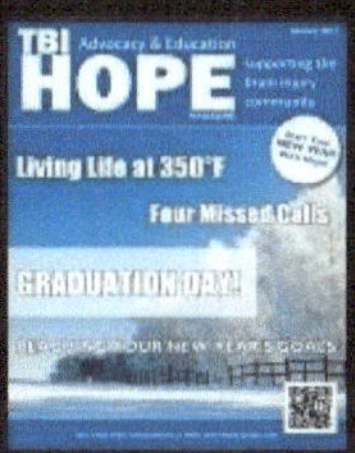
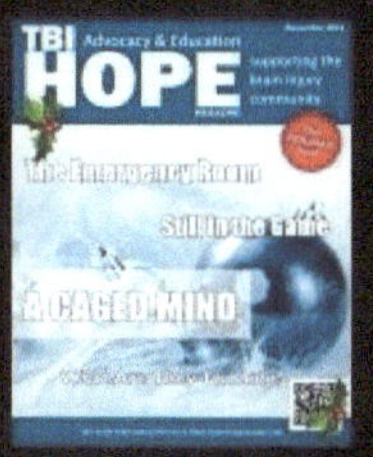
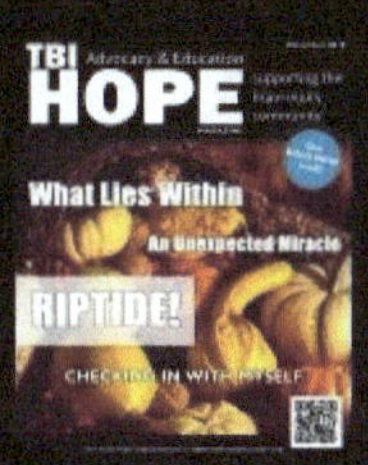
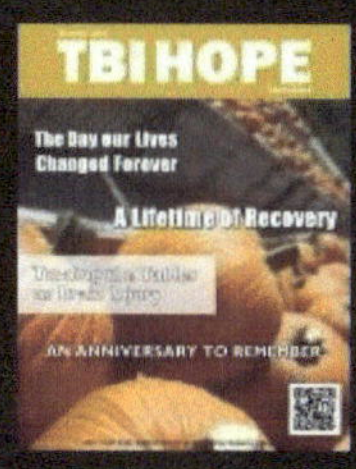
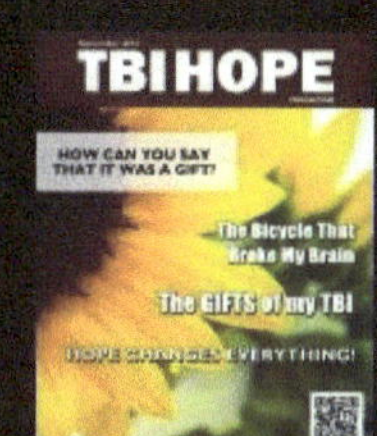
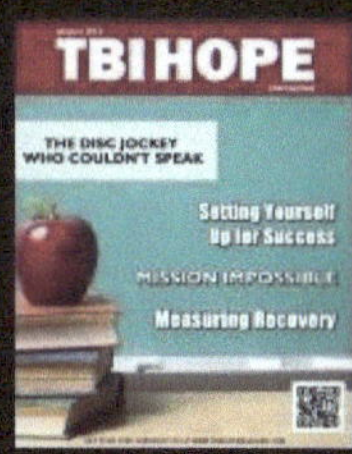
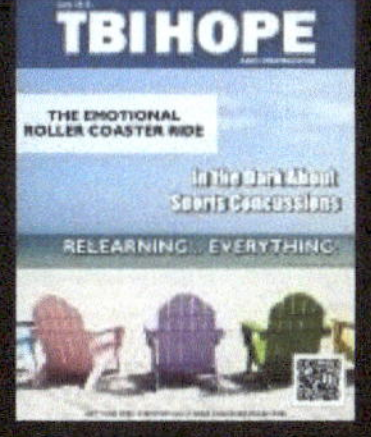
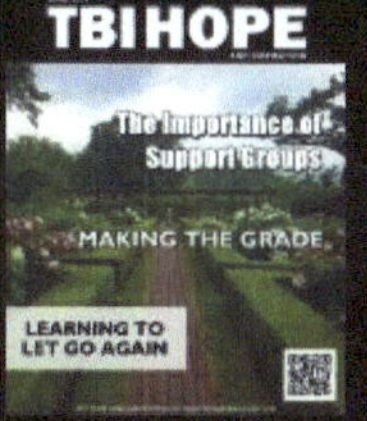
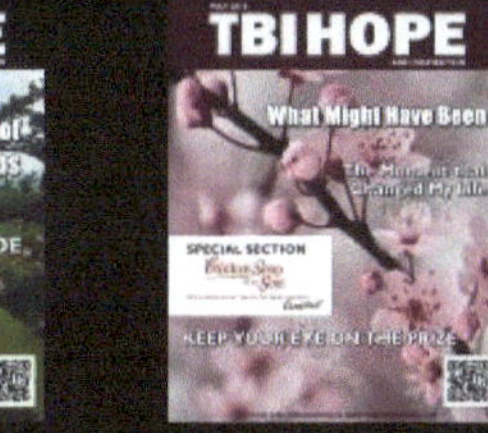
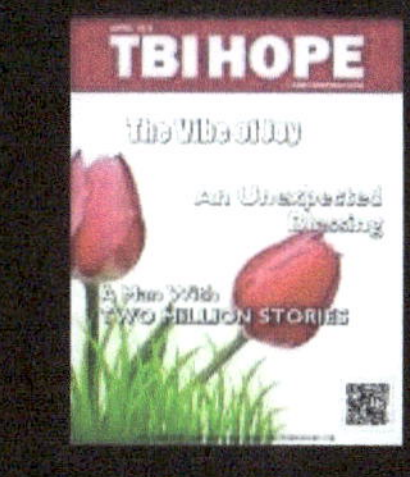
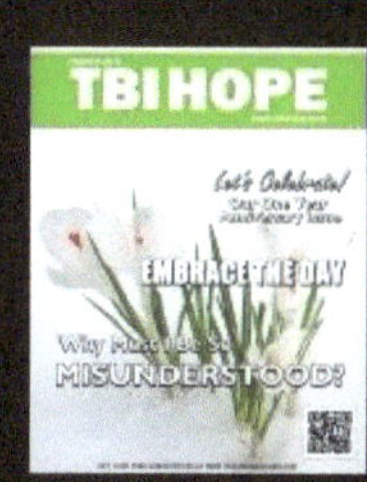
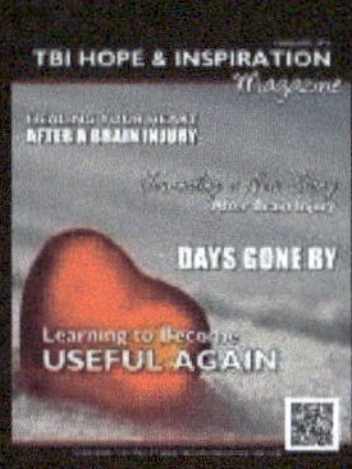
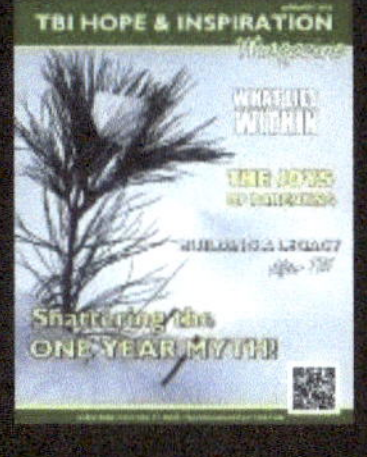
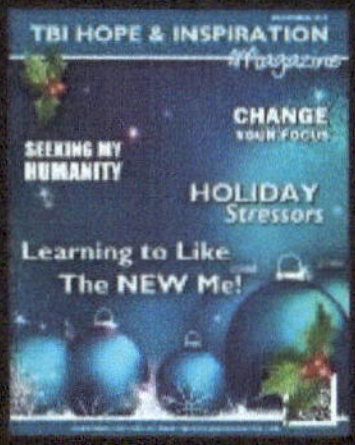
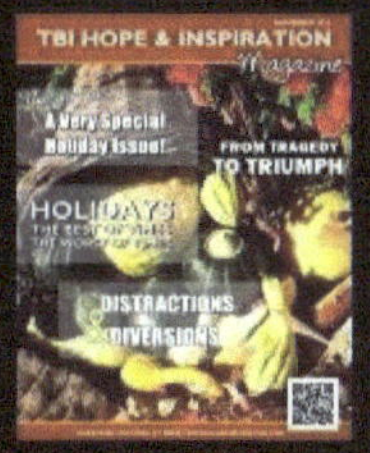
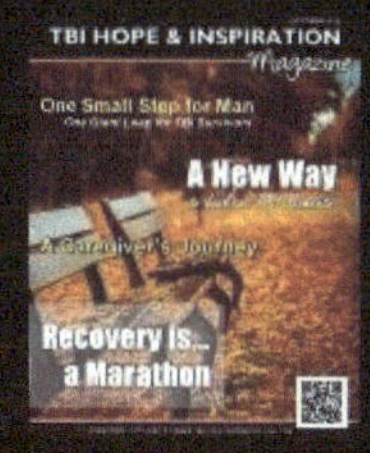
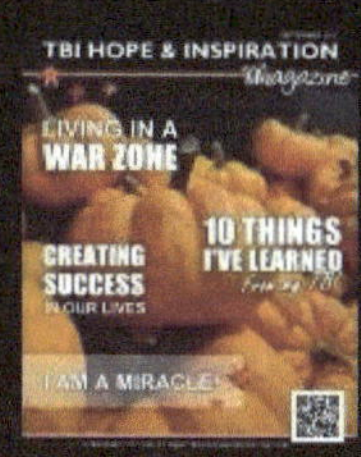
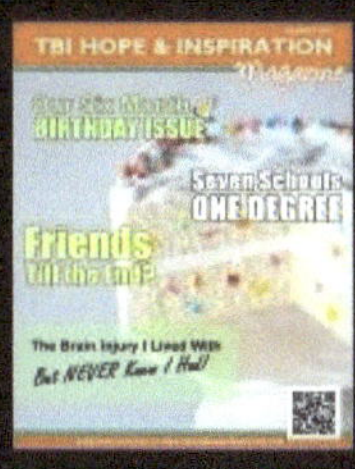
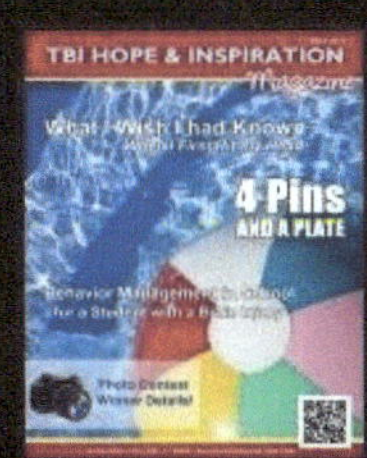
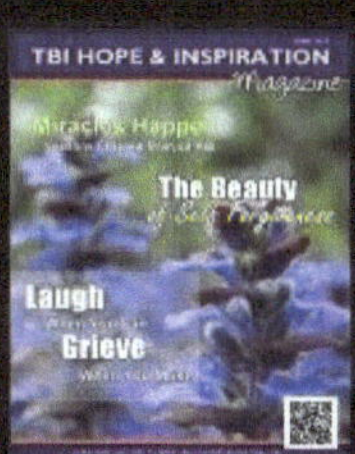
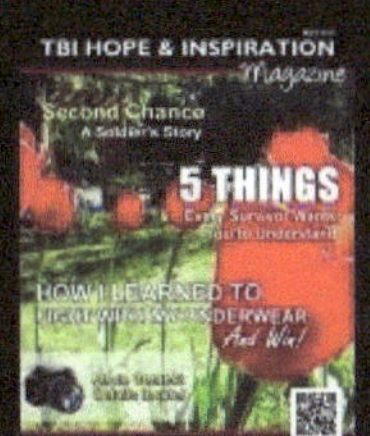
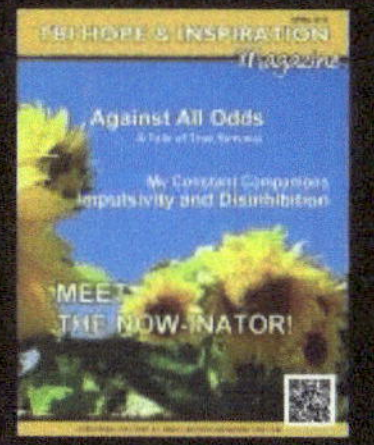
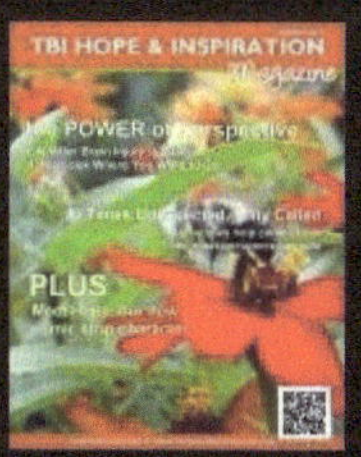

HOPE MAGAZINE

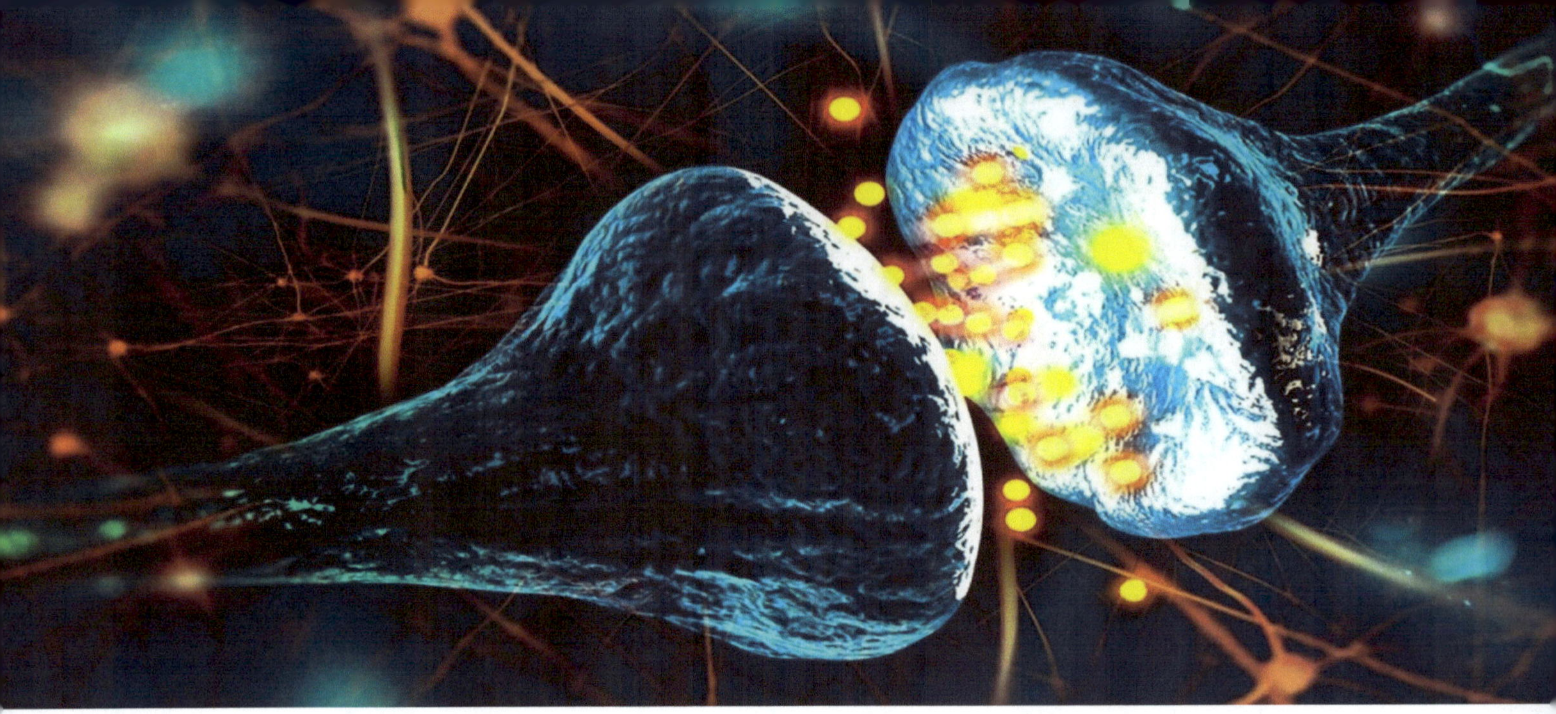

Keeping the Faith
By Kellie Pokrifka

It's not that I was suicidal. No – that's so active; so intentional. But, maybe? A little bit, sure. I mean, yeah, just don't tell anybody. So uncomfortable. No, that's not *me*.

It was mostly me alternating between two images. The first would be if I did not do anything. *Do anything, do something* – my innocuous little euphemism concealing any trace that I considered murdering myself. If I did not *do something,* I would wake up twenty years later and still be in the same position: in excruciating pain, helpless, lying in my childhood bedroom, wistfully remembering when I thought I would finish college, and might even finish medical school. You know, to really have something to show and really be able to help people. In that image in my mind, I would regret not taking action before then. Why did I prolong this suffering? I knew nothing was going to result from my life after Traumatic Brain Injury.

> My innocuous little euphemism was concealing any trace that I considered murdering myself.

And then I would force myself into jumping to the second image – the image if I actually *did* do something. It was my little brother, the sunshine of my life, trembling while he stands over my coffin, and the devastation that would occur for either one of us to go on without the other. He stands over me, his pale blue eyes drenched and bloodshot, absorbing the weight that he was not enough to make me stay. The weight of the realization that his hero just up and quit on life.

That image felt so much worse than the first, so that image always won.

I kept on, every day, assuming that each following day would be equally as devastating. But that assumption was just another lie that my injury was telling me. So many malfunctions in my body manifested as these thoughts. My gut decayed itself in the aftermath of the injury, and that's where 95% of serotonin, the happy hormone, is produced. This depletion presented itself as this harrowing depression. A substantial amount of dopamine also originates in the gut. Dopamine serves as the foundation for the reward pathway. When something good happens, dopamine makes you want to do that action again. A depletion of dopamine serves as the basis for TBI patients losing all interest in activities which we used to treasure.

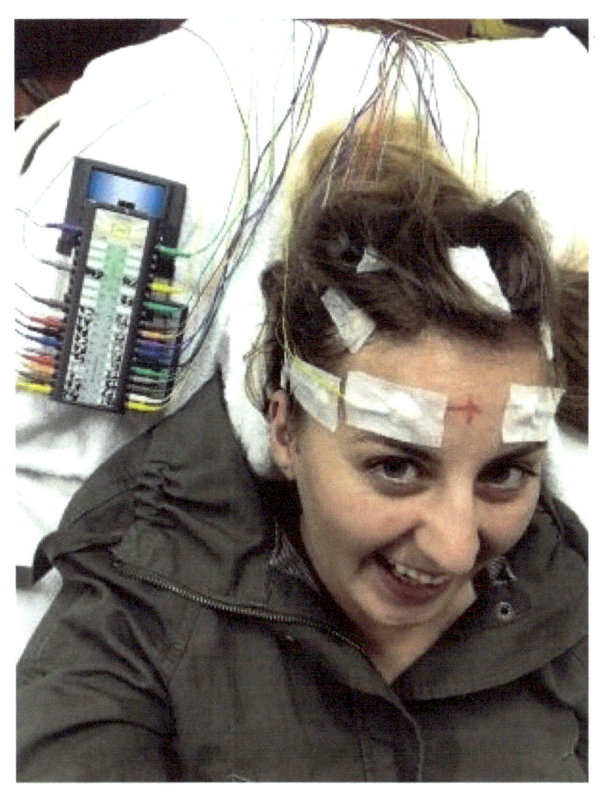

Also, like one third of all TBI patients, pituitary dysfunction forced my hormonal system to spiral out of control. The countless bodily processes regulated by hormones were now also dictated by malfunctioning messages. Sleep all day; rage over a minor agitation; feel emotionally distraught over nothing. These messages were not reality for me, and you should know it is not reality for you either. Our brain injuries shout over us, drowning out all of our reason and all of our organic personalities.

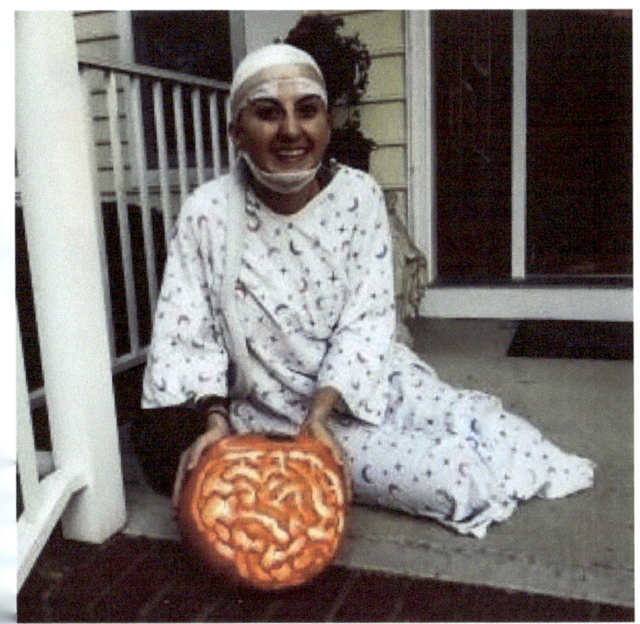

Recovery will mute these horrendous messages. Your real voice will return. You just need to hold on and have hope and faith in your body's ability to heal.

You need to seek out the treatment methods designed for your specific symptoms. This can amount to needle-in-a-haystack levels of impossible. But that treatment is out there, waiting to bring you back to *you.* You will encounter more than enough naysayers along your journey who hold no right to interfere with your progress. Leave them to complain by themselves.

You need to abandon every doctor who does not believe in your recovery and does not painstakingly strive towards that goal. You, and only you, can conquer the battle that is your brain. But a few consistent cheerleaders always lighten the burden.

Today, the same agonizing pain I endured during that time period still exists and still plagues me each day. But now, this pain stands as the only thing I have to battle – those thoughts have cleared. My chemicals no longer lie to me. My body finally allied along with me to win this war. Never have I been more grateful for my life than I am right now. But looking back, those thoughts never originated from me not trying hard enough to be grateful. I was trying so hard and fighting so hard every single day. Never was it a personality flaw. It was the injury. These injuries can be healed. Have faith in that.

Meet Kellie Pokrifka

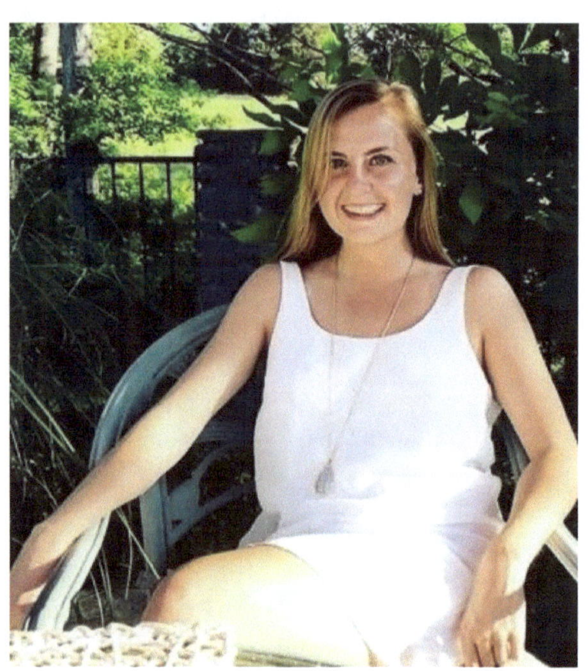

Kellie Pokrifka experienced a Traumatic Brain Injury at age 19. This immediately forced her to take medical leave from the University of Virginia. Her doctors continued to give her timelines of recovery, and yet the injury progressively worsened. Four years later, she still experiences a wide array of symptoms. Throughout her journey, she realized how little information on brain injury recovery is publically available. Doctors tend to preach the 'rest and wait' method when so many more effective therapies go unrecognized. Kellie has taken this very personal cause and works to compile the latest research on TBI therapies and make it available to those in need. Follow her on Instagram @concusssiongameplan. No brain injury survivor should have to fight so hard to hear about therapy options.

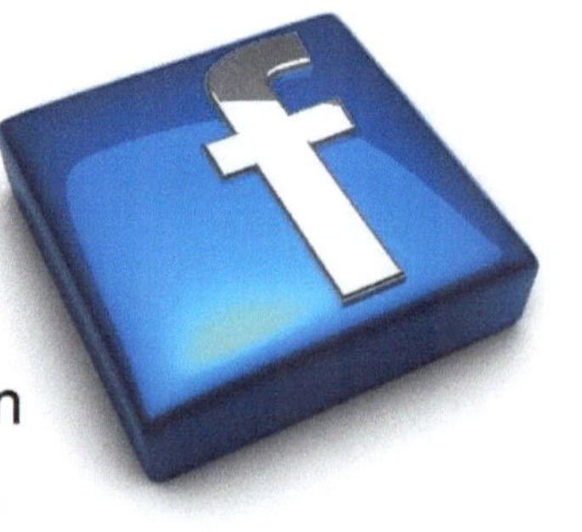

Finding Senior Housing can be complex, but it doesn't have to be.

Call A Place for Mom. Our Advisors are trusted, local experts who can help you understand your options. Since 2000, we've helped over one million families find senior living solutions that meet their unique needs.

"You can trust **A Place for Mom** to help you."

– *Joan Lunden*

a Place *for* Mom.

A Free Service for Families.
Call: (844) 578-9504

A Place for Mom is the nation's largest senior living referral information service. We do not own, operate, endorse or recommend any senior living community. We are paid by partner communities, so our services are completely free to families.

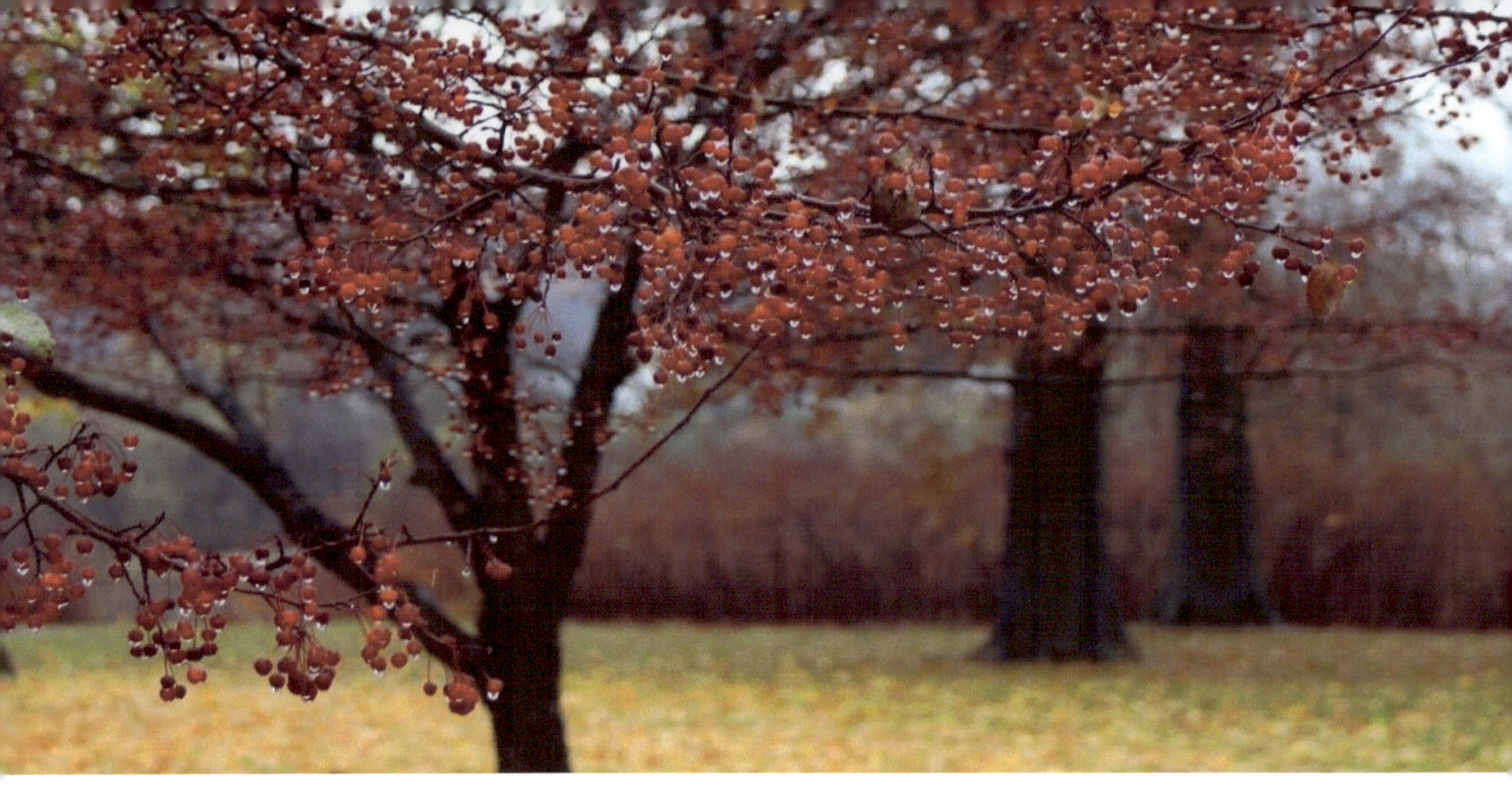

A Servant's Heart
By Connie Zanoni

Tuesday June 10, 2008, was a beautiful, sunny day and the sky was cobalt blue with not a cloud in sight. As I drove home from work that night, I was talking to God about my perfect life. My son was married and in the Coast Guard, I had a smart and beautiful new daughter in law, my daughter was in college and on the dean's list, my husband and I were happily married for 27 years, I had just gotten a new car and I was finally working at my dream job. We were all healthy and we still had our parents. I closed my prayer with, "Thank You Lord, I finally have it all." I will never repeat those words as long as I live.

Three days later, Friday, June 13, was Yard Sale Day. My daughter and I were up early and shared some special vanilla coffee. We had prepared for our yard sale for days, because all of the proceeds would buy more books for her education. Everything was going as planned and then I saw a box that we missed. I pulled it backwards and was caught off-guard by how heavy it was. Then I lost my footing. As I began to free fall, the back of my head collided with a log splitter. Life changed drastically in a second and it was terrifying.

> As I began to free fall, the back of my head collided with a log splitter. Life changed drastically in a second and it was terrifying.

I lost the dream job and the car. My husband faced struggles that would have made most men walk away. My daughter didn't see a glimmer of her beautiful, talented, funny and patient Mom. But there was and is always hope. I could go on about all the struggles of Traumatic Brain Injury but you all know those well enough.

My story is about progress and taking what is left, making it enough and then multiplying that into abundant joy. My story is about relearning a modest skill which gave me tremendous hope that established a series of events to take place. This hope continues to be so beneficial to me that nearly ten years later, this basic, relearned skill still calms me down, brings me focus and helps me to give back to others.

I was born with a servant's heart but since my brain injury I am lucky to get breakfast for myself. Therapists came into my home several days a week. Many people helped me with my daily tasks. I slept a lot and I felt like a worthless burden. I could not drive a car. Lights and noise seemed to destruct me like a bomb on a battlefield. An old friend came to visit me about six months after my accident. While

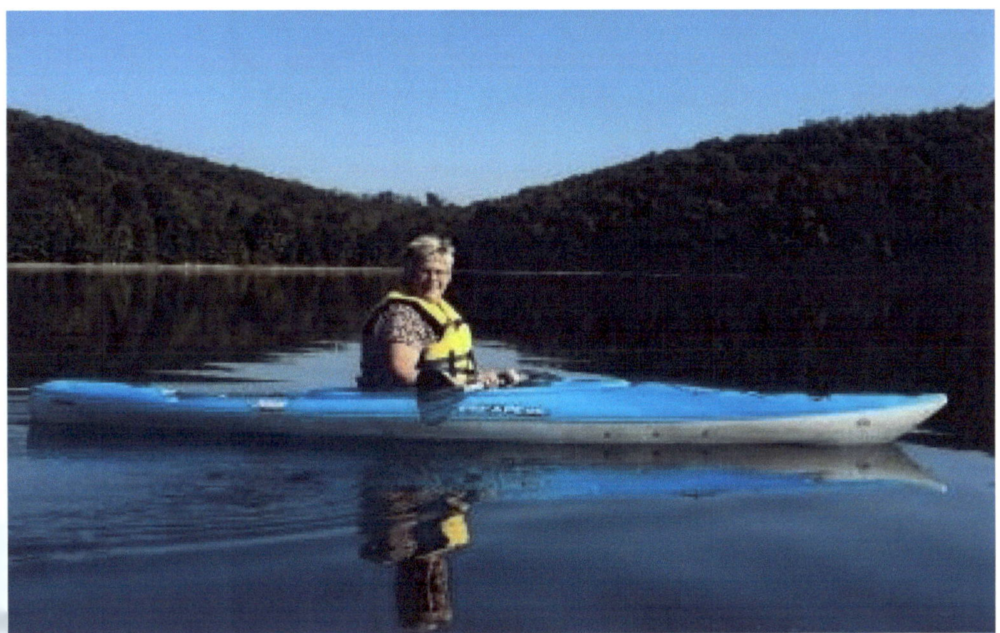

sitting on my porch one evening, she suggested that I try to make prayer shawls. She knew I had knitted and crocheted before the accident. In the beginning, I was filled with frustration and inadequacy. I could not remember how to cast on stitches, and following the pattern was out of the question. I crumbled up the pattern and threw my yarn aside, feeling defeated. My friend did not give up on me. She came to my home repeatedly and helped me relearn one basic crochet stitch. I crocheted, she ripped out my stitch, and I got angry. I struggled, but with determination I repeated that one stitch again and again. It began to look neater and eventually I created prayer shawls. I was finally able to give back in the quiet privacy of my own home. A sense of purpose flooded my soul.

Then, my daughter saw a cute teddy bear hat pattern. She remembered my skills before the brain injury and encouraged me to try it out. Together we found a pattern using the same stitch I'd learned, and sure enough. I made a simple but cute hat from that pattern with little effort. Hats were done rather quickly so my attention was kept better than with a shawl. Today, I continue to crochet hats for three local school districts. They give away the hats to students who don't have any.

My 83-year-old Mom continued to encourage me to interact with others. When I finally began to drive again, I formed a group at my church appropriately called, "Humble Hands." We are a group of women ranging from 55 to 93 who meet every week. Together we sew, cut, crochet and stretch our limits with new projects. We make knotted quilts for a nursing home and a children's aid home, dementia fidget blankets for Alzheimer's patients, prayer shawls, hats, gloves, and mittens for local schools.

So…you're going through a rough time, believe me, I GET that! I can tell you that it is not the end of your world, it is merely a detour. Sometimes detours are short, while other times they take you miles and miles around and the ride is long. Try to enjoy the scenery. Be careful of those speed bumps! When you are tired, pull over and rest. Try your hardest to enjoy this detour because the old road may never reopen. Like me, you may remain on the new detour but I am certain you can be better than you were yesterday. I am still not making any knitted cable sweaters but I am adding JOY to my life by giving back to others! A vital part of your recovery is to find a small way to give back. You need to look past yourself to others. Do not ever give up on yourself and continue to test your abilities.

Meet Connie Zanoni

I am a wife to a supportive man, Mom to a son and daughter and Oma to four amazing grandchildren. I enjoy walking, gardening, writing, singing and any craft. Living with a traumatic brain injury has its challenges but I try to find joy in each day and have learned the importance of stepping out of my comfort zone.

Bright Red Berries Holding Onto Rain

I was in the summer of my life
Blue skies and sunshine left me warm and radiant
My abundant fruits were seen everywhere
6.13.08 Traumatic Brain Injury
Seasons changed and now I am like
A cold gray autumn day
With bright red berries holding onto rain, like tears
Yet even on a cold gray autumn day
Skills slowly appear, just like bright gold leaves
Accomplishments shine like red berries and
Side effects like rainy tears can blur my mind
Yet I can see beauty in me, beauty in traumatic brain injury
Like a cold gray autumn day
With bright red berries holding onto rain
I can see beauty
Can you see beauty?

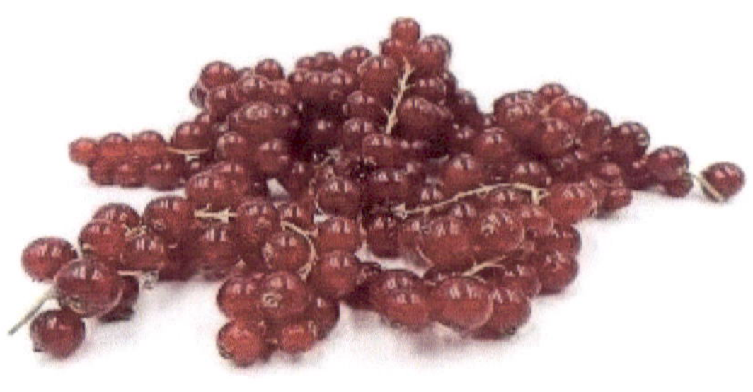

A poem written by Connie for a Traumatic Brain Injury Voices Project.

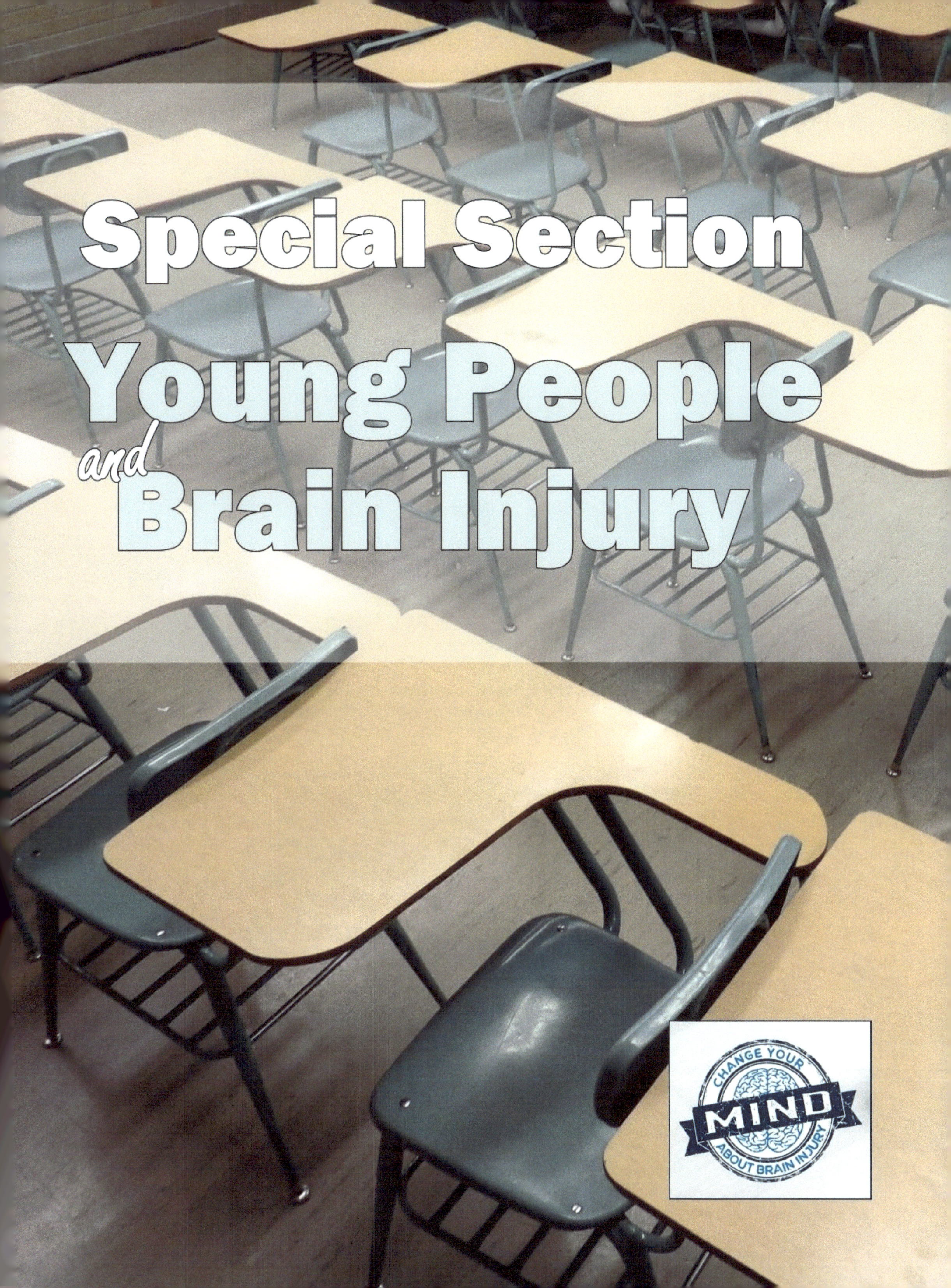
Special Section
Young People
and
Brain Injury
CHANGE YOUR
MIND
ABOUT BRAIN INJURY

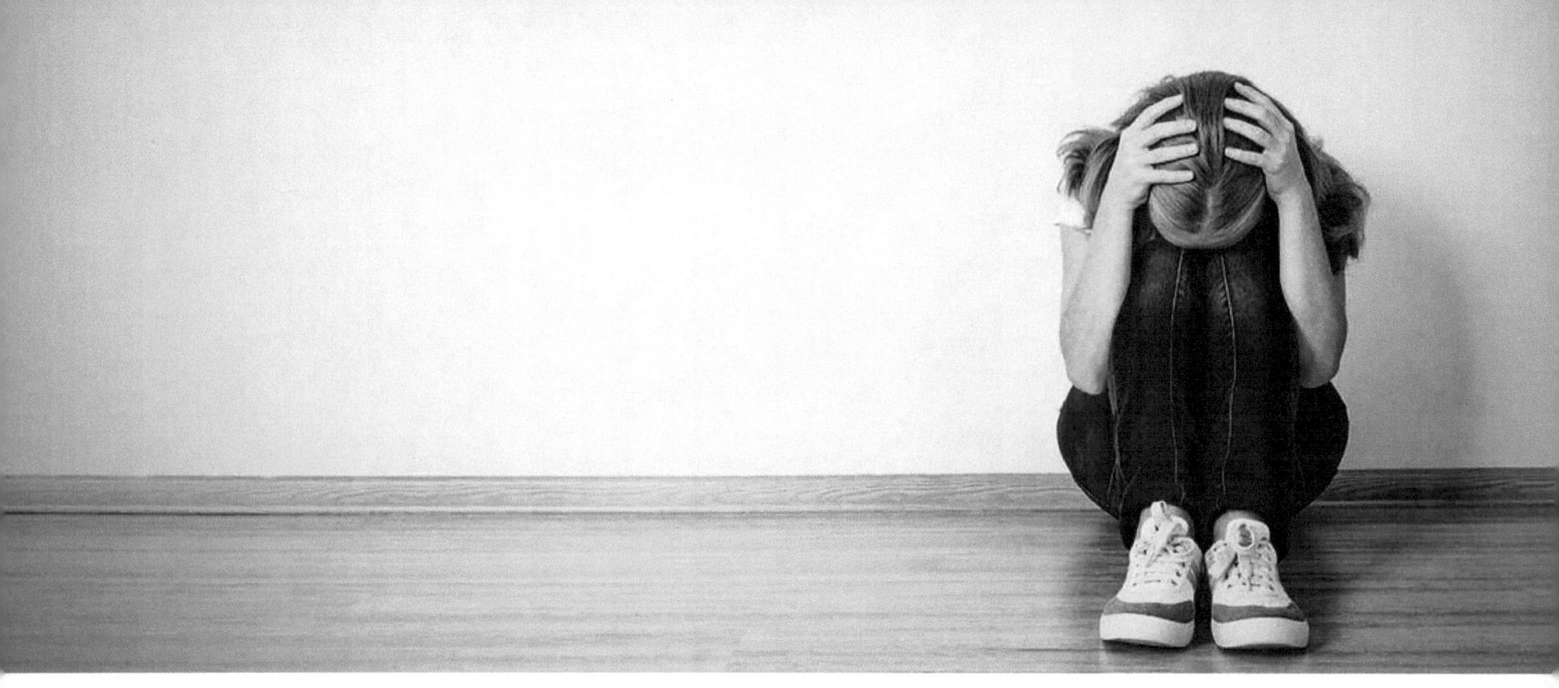

Returning to Life

By Haley Anderson

My TBI occurred during the spring break of my junior year of high school, in 2014. Before my injury, I had been an honors student taking college-level classes, I participated in five clubs on campus, and I was a member of the Pep Band, Jazz Band, Wind Ensemble, and was also in the pit orchestra for my school's musicals. My bubbly personality and bright smile lit up a room and I brought warmth to the lives of those around me.

After my accident, I had trouble walking and talking, I had tunnel vision for nearly a year, and my short- and long-term memory were shot. I got intense motion sickness when I rode in the car for longer than ten minutes, if I turned my head too fast, or if I stood up too fast. I had a headache all day every day for months on end, I was extremely sensitive to light and sound, and I put on more than 30 pounds due to various medications and inactivity. I spent the three months following my injury curled up in a ball in my room because I was in so much pain. I had nightmares every night for more than a year and I suffered from post-concussive syndrome, anxiety, and depression. I became sullen and quiet and struggled to find joy in the things that had previously made me so happy.

> I spent the three months following my injury curled up in a ball in my room because I was in so much pain.

For reasons listed above, I was not able to return to school that year and did not finish my junior year of high school. When I returned to school the next year for my senior year, I wasn't sure if I was going to be able to graduate on time. Fortunately, because I had been such a high achiever in the previous years, I only needed to complete one class to fulfill the requirements for graduation. I graduated from high school in June of 2015 and started school at the local community college in September, later that year.

Starting college while recovering from a head injury was a daunting task for my parents and doctors and they advised me to take it slow. However, I—being the stubborn, high-achieving perfectionist that I am—wanted to jump in at full speed. We all compromised and decided that I would start the quarter with two classes equaling five credits. I was in denial about how bad my condition was and had convinced myself that I would be fine.

What a slap in the face the first week was. Everything that I used to do with ease (focusing in class, taking notes, keeping up with homework, remembering facts, figures, and readings from my textbook) was impossible. Despite my challenges I've managed to do well in my classes over the past three years—receiving A's and B's—but the thing I struggled with the most was the realization that everything I had been able to do was dramatically altered. Working through that realization was one of the hardest things I have had to do throughout this journey and it took some time for me to adjust and to figure out how to work around my challenges.

Working with the disability center at school was incredibly helpful to me during my first two years of college. I received accommodations in the classroom (such as priority seating in the front of the class), I took my tests in a quiet room, and I received double time on all my tests and quizzes. Over the last year, I have made great strides in my recovery. I lost the 30 pounds I had put on in the first year, I hardly ever use the disability center at school now, and I recently dropped the last medication I was taking for my TBI. Keeping active has become incredibly important to me. In November I ran my first half-marathon and in January I joined a cross-fit gym.

I am currently in my third year of attending the local community college. I just completed the last of the classes needed for my associate's degree and am now working on completing prerequisites for nursing school. After I have completed nursing school, I hope to join the U.S. Navy and work as a nurse on the hospital ship USNS Mercy or USNS Comfort doing humanitarian work overseas. This summer, I will be traveling to Indonesia for two weeks for a combined study abroad / volunteer trip where I will be distributing eyeglasses and The Shoe That Grows to the locals in Bali and Java with my classmates.

Looking back at the struggles I had to face every day makes me incredibly proud to be where I am today, and I know that things can only go up from here!

Meet Haley Anderson

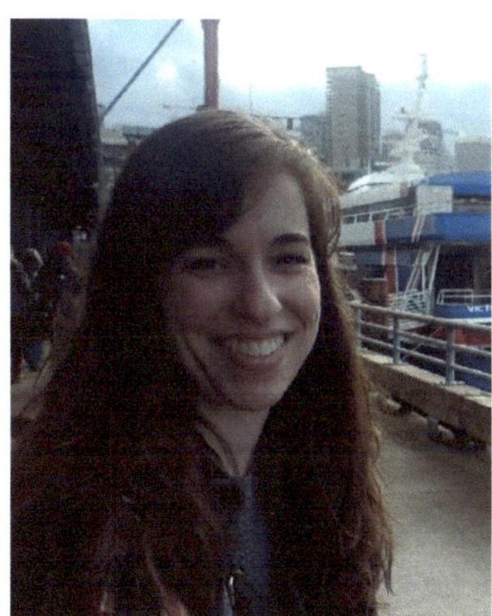

Haley Anderson is a 21-year-old college student currently living in Washington State and is four years post-injury. She enjoys hiking, CrossFit, painting, rowing, and camping and spending time with family and friends. Haley always has a smile on her face and her happy personality is infectious. She has faced all the challenges that life has thrown at her with grace and dignity and has not let her brain injury deter her from her goals.

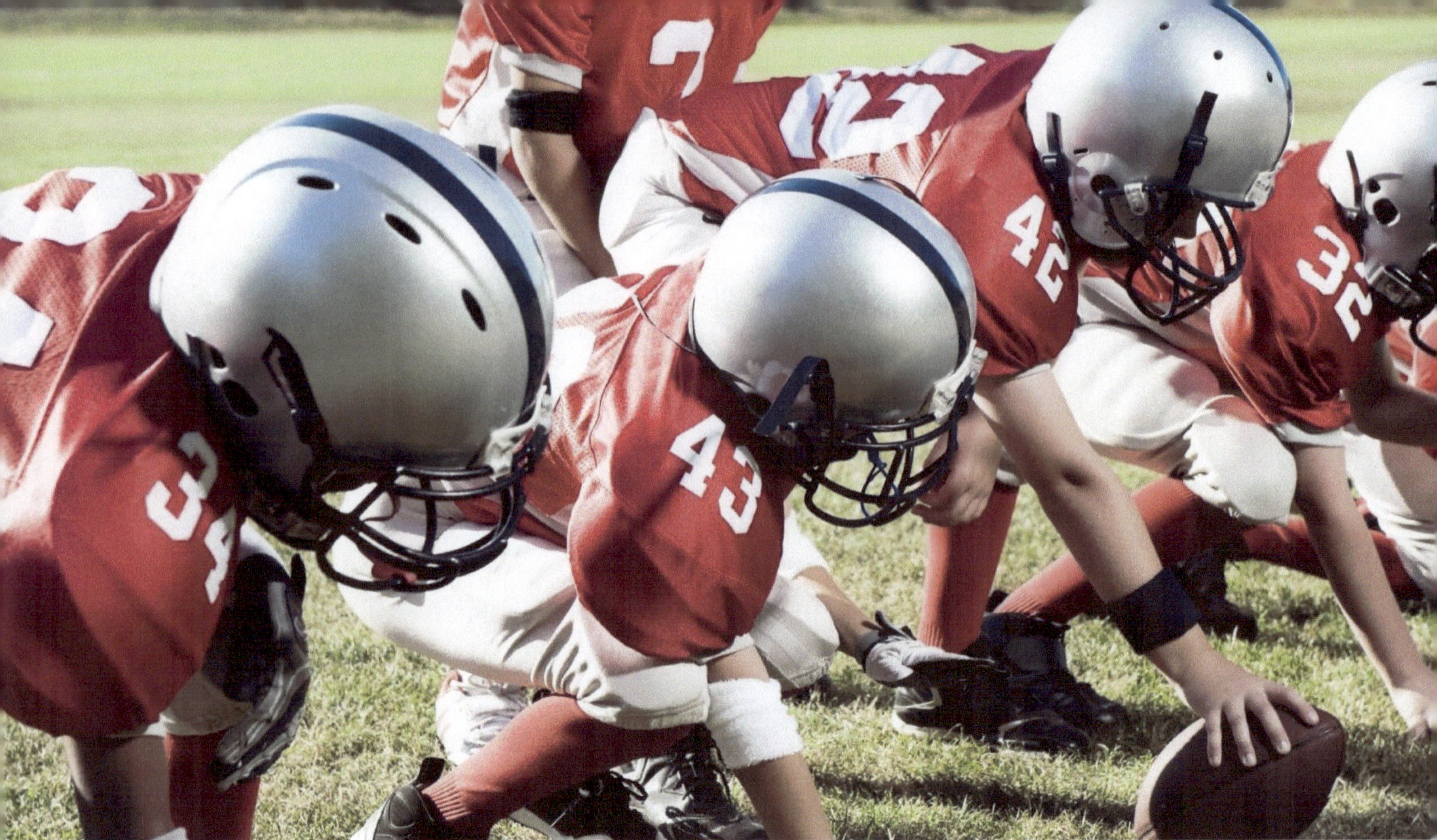

I AM TBI
By Adam Hapworth

Most of the stories I read are about how a Traumatic Brain Injury changes someone's life after their accident or injury. Like how it made them different from the way they were before. What if you didn't fully know or have realized who you were, or were to become, before TBI happened to you? What if it happened during a time when the term Traumatic Brain Injury wasn't common nomenclature and the effects were not mainstream news? Here is my story about how my TBI a month after my 15th birthday may have changed my life.

In 1992, I was a freshman in high school playing my first year of organized football. I had always played in the front yard or sandlot with my friends. As tough teens we didn't need any pads or protection, just the ability to take or, preferably, give a big hit and get up. I may have given myself any number of mild head injuries during that time. In the '80's and '90's if you were not puking or passed out, a headache wasn't a big deal.

For about half of the season, I had gained the admiration of the coaches for how hard I worked and played and with that they had me in nearly every play all game long. I was offense as a tight end, defense as a middle linebacker, and on special teams. I took every opportunity to prove I had what it took to be a reliable football player.

During our last game of the season against the rival neighboring team, I was playing on defense with my team mates and after one play, nothing of special remembrance, we got into a defense huddle and my head started pounding. I waved over to the coach letting him know I was coming out. When I got to him I told him my head was pounding and he had me head over to the bench to rest for a bit. That is the last thing I remember about the game.

> **I had suffered a Subdural Hematoma with a blood clot on the brain. As I was going to sit on the bench during the game, I collapsed to the ground had a seizure, and stopped breathing.**

I woke up and noticed a hazy shadow of a TV. I was confused, because I didn't have a TV in my room. I reached to scratch my head and felt something there. I took what looked like a turban of gauze off into my hands. Freaking out, I hurried to put it back on, finally noticing I was in the hospital. I had been there for three days, unknown to me.

I had suffered a Subdural Hematoma with a blood clot on the brain. As I was going to sit on the bench during the game, I collapsed to the ground had a seizure, and stopped breathing. The athletic trainer rushed over while the ambulance staff at the end of the field – uncommon at the time – rushed in to get me loaded and off to the hospital. I have heard that I woke halfway through the surgery and started pulling tubes out; none of it is in my memory, just an imagination of what it might have looked like.

Again, this was in 1992. After I woke up, I could walk and talk and seemed to be my normal teenage self, just a bit weak and weary from what had occurred. I stayed for observation for another four days. I was released and went home for another week to rest, before going back to school. During that time my mother took me for what I would call a cognitive test. It was basically a paper test of shapes and sentences and repetition to see how well I could remember and think. I believe I passed it, I never really knew.

Back then, there was no talk of how TBI would affect you as a person, no talk of depression, possible memory issues, and behavior changes. Truthfully, there was no talk of TBI. The only related appointment to my head injury was the cognitive test. On all outside appearances I was the same 15-year-old boy who had gotten lucky and not died. But was I?

My best friend had always been the people person, and I was the quiet one who always had fun. I was the upbeat wisecracking goofball guy, nicknamed "Happy," (after my last name of Hapworth, and my behavior). But inside, I was fighting depression, though I didn't know it at the time, because it wasn't talked about. I didn't want to do school work. I just wanted to live in the moment. Keeping focus on one thing for a long time just wasn't possible. These were all normal teenage behaviors, right?

I graduated from high school with average grades and went to college to study Computer Information Systems. Computers were the one thing I could concentrate on. In 1998, during my second year of college, I met a beautiful woman who, in less than a year, became my loving wife and we had a child together shortly after. We went through a rough spell around 2005. I wasn't being the best husband, and I was in the grips of a very deep depression. I didn't want to do anything and, at that time, we had two kids under five years of old. I went to counseling and was prescribed medication for my depression. About six months later, I felt like a completely different person. I weaned myself off the meds and I felt human again.

Since then, I have been doing well as a computer programmer. Now, through reading and understanding the complexity of the human mind and its relation to TBI, I am seeing signs of things that many other people may not notice or have to deal with: the lack of focus, memory issues, social anxieties, and bouts of depression. Now, I am a forty-year-old father of four, having had a TBI for 26 years of my life, and my memory is starting to be worrisome; concerns over CTE are creeping in as well.

My TBI happened at an age where the definition of who I would become as a person was just beginning. The former me was just a child. Some days I still feel as if I am a fifteen-year-old boy in forty-year-old skin. My TBI made me who I am, and right now I am very happy with who that is.

Meet Adam Hapworth

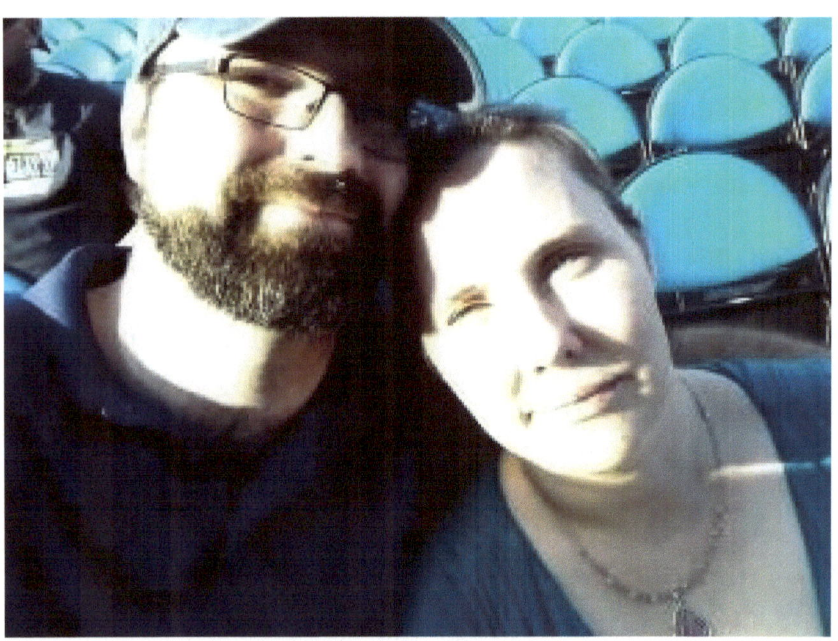

In 1992, Adam suffered a subdural hematoma and blood clot on the brain on his high school football field. Today, Adam lives in Clinton, Maine, next door to where he grew up, with his wife of nineteen years, and their four children. Their oldest child is going to Wheaton college majoring in neuroscience.

After Adam's injury, he completed high school and then went on to college. He received a Bachelor's Degree in computer information systems and has been employed as a computer programmer for almost twenty years.

Adam says, "In 1992, a head injury, in my opinion, was misunderstood. Either you died, became visibly disabled (speech or motion defects), or you were just fine. I fell back into the "just fine." For me now, reading studies and other survivors' stories, I understand that the reasons I was depressed or have focus and memory issues may not just be a normal course of growing up for me. I'm at the point in my life where I'd like to give back and help others in a similar situation."

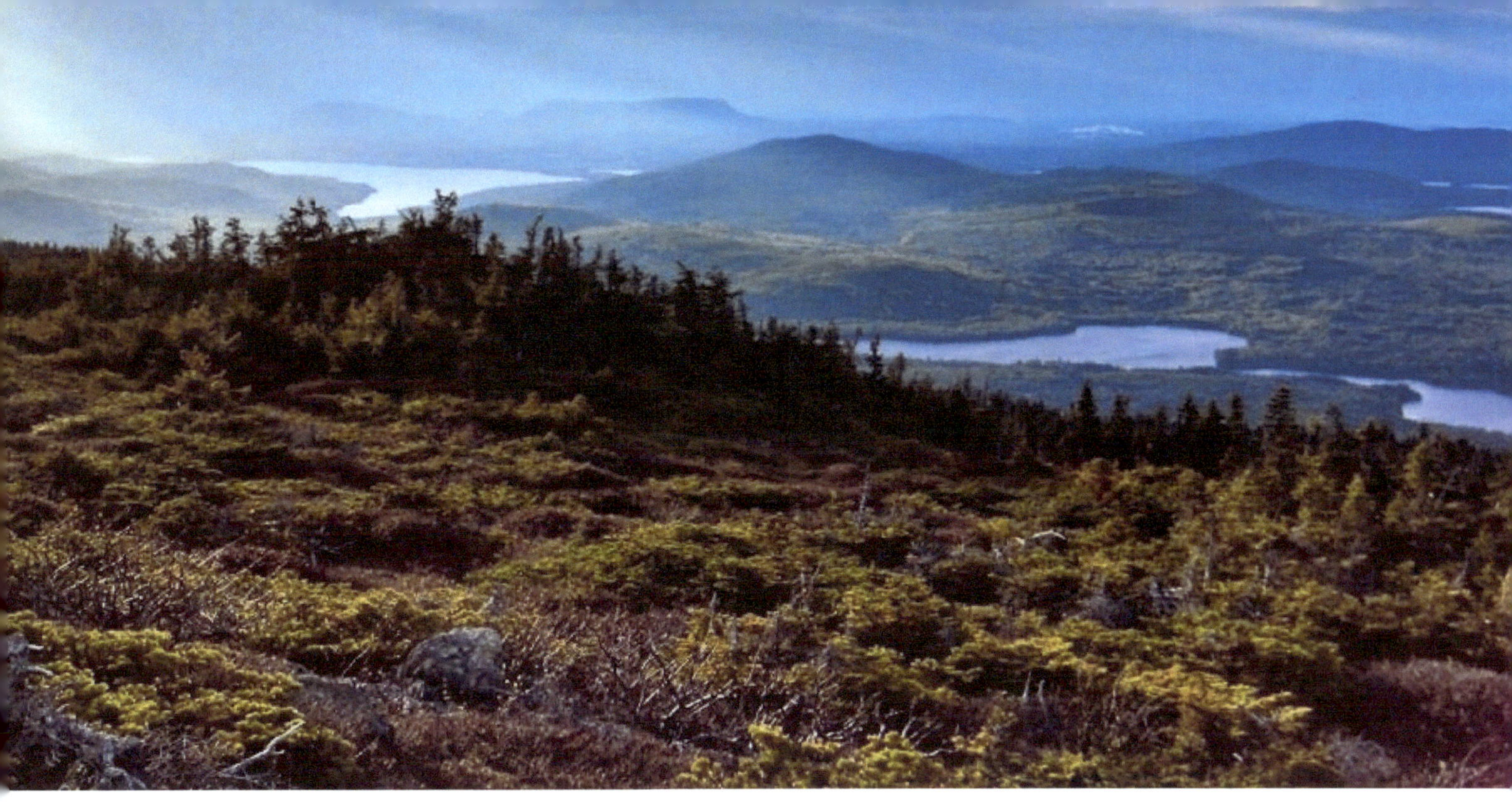

Overcoming Barriers
By Sarah Kilch Gaffney

I was fourteen or fifteen years old when I got my first concussion and nineteen when I received my last, amassing approximately eight in the intervening years. This occurred before we knew much about the cumulative nature of head injuries and before we paid much attention to them, and the last one was where they all caught up with me.

In my final college soccer game, I collided with a player from the opposing team. The details are fuzzy, but ultimately her knee connected directly under my chin. I was stunned and it took a few minutes to get me off the field. Sitting on the sideline, I took off my goalkeeper gloves and, realizing I had forgotten my mouth guard that day, palpated my jaw, grateful that my teeth were still intact.

> When I finally saw a doctor over a week later, I was told I had classic concussion symptoms.

My tongue swelled and the student athletic trainer crushed up something so that I could swallow it. The next day, I was exhausted and in pain. My parents, both former EMTs, wanted me to be evaluated. When I brought up my continued symptoms, the athletic director told me that I did not need an evaluation and I certainly did not have a concussion because "he saw concussions every day in football."

When I finally saw a doctor over a week later I was told I had classic concussion symptoms. After weeks of sleeping nearly twenty hours a day, taking incompletes in all of my classes that term, and months of headaches and medications, I eventually recovered. I stopped playing soccer and swore off activities that might easily result in another knock to the head.

The following summer, I decided to serve as an AmeriCorps volunteer on a backcountry trail crew in the Maine wilderness. There, on a mountain on the Appalachian Trail, I met Steve, a tall, lanky fellow from northern Vermont. Less than two years later, on a bright October day, Steve and I were married on that same mountain.

Shortly after our third wedding anniversary, Steve and I arrived back at our car after a weekend hike, and he couldn't speak. First there was silence, then gibberish, then real words but in no logical order, then it was as if nothing at all had happened. He was completely back to himself and assured me he was fine.

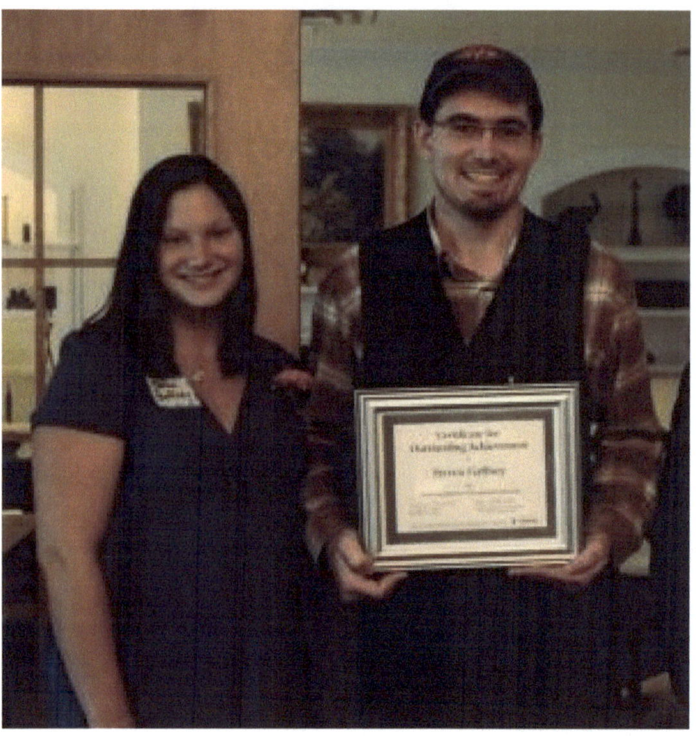

Steve receiving Maine General's Overcoming Barriers Award in 2010.

The following day, Steve was diagnosed with a massive brain tumor. He was 27 years old.

Steve was a champion of patience and humor, attributes that had served him well in his work teaching others how to build trails, and he held onto his good nature and easy-going attitude as we faced an uncertain future.

He joked, laughed, and smiled his way through two awake brain surgeries, radiation, multiple chemotherapies, and proton beam radiation. I can't count the number of times we walked down the halls of his cancer center hand in hand with me in tears and him telling me it was going to be okay.

When he awoke from the first brain surgery with cognitive and speech challenges, Steve dove head first into speech therapy, earning himself an *"Overcoming Barriers"* award from our local hospital. When the radiation therapy left him permanently disabled, he maintained his positive outlook. When he became homebound during the last few months of his life, he was still able to smile – a fact for which I will always be extremely grateful and in absolute awe of.

Shortly after his diagnosis, Steve's oncologist had revealed to us that his tumor would eventually be terminal, and we tried our best to live our life while carrying that knowledge. Along the way, our daughter was born, and Steve loved her with absolutely everything he had.

Steve's doctors never talked about brain injuries. Though, of course, that is what he was experiencing, over and over again. His oncologist was concerned with the efficacy of chemotherapy, his neurosurgeon with the delicate balance of cutting too much versus too little, his neurologist with controlling his seizures. And, so, no one talked about brain injuries, or what to expect, or where to seek help, support, or information. We didn't even talk to a social worker until the week before Steve started hospice.

Until the last couple weeks of his life, Steve had little pain. His fatigue, however, was immense and unrelenting. Everything made him tired and each new treatment increased the weight of that burden, building over the years.

As treatments failed and his tumor progressed, Steve slowly lost cognitive and physical function. Eventually, he could no longer walk, no longer leave the house, and then no longer leave the hospital bed that we had squeezed into our bedroom.

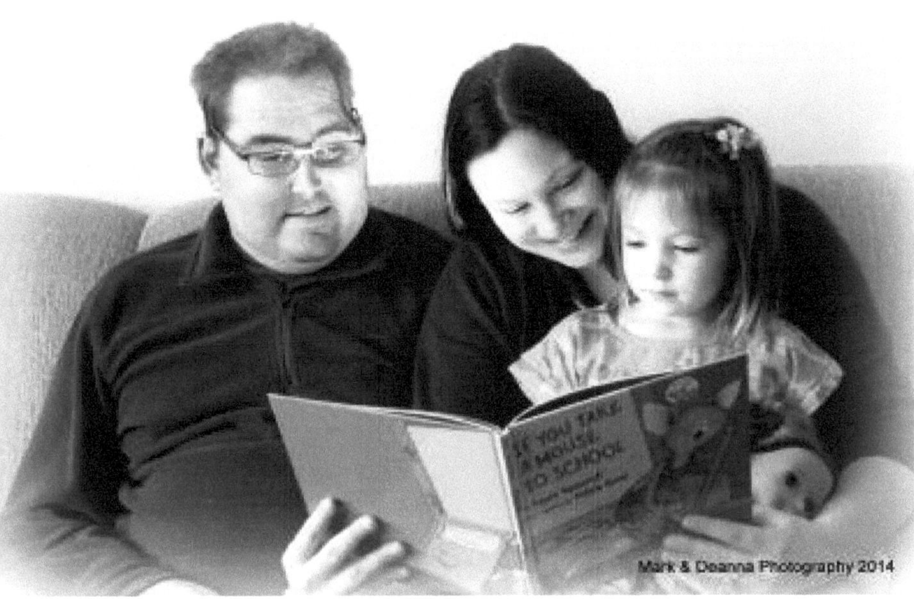

The family together shortly after Steve started hospice.

Steve died at home two months shy of his 32nd birthday, four and a half years after his diagnosis. I found myself reeling, widowed with a toddler, and with no idea what to do or how to make my way through life now that Steve was no longer by my side.

When Steve became disabled, I had started working towards nursing school. We had both continued to work in the conservation field after we met, but I felt that I now needed a different career to support our family. I fought hard to follow through with that decision, juggling Steve's treatments and care with raising our daughter, work, school, and managing a house.

I left nursing school to take care of Steve during the last months of his life, and returned after he died, but despite my 4.0 GPA and outward success, I was miserable and it became clear that it was no longer where I needed to be. At the time, it seemed hard to believe that there would ever be another right path, but I desperately needed a change and a break.

I didn't take much of a break, but I did find the change that I needed. A little over a year after Steve's death and just over a month after I left nursing school, I accepted a position as the Program Coordinator for the Brain Injury Association of America's Maine Chapter. It's a dream job, and I still sometimes pinch myself to make sure it's real.

Now, I get to spend my days increasing awareness about brain injury, helping survivors and families get the resources and support that they need, and being an

> **I accepted a position as the Program Coordinator for the Brain Injury Association of America's Maine Chapter.**

important voice for those with brain injury in Maine. I get to provide the support that didn't exist when Steve was sick, and I get to make sure survivors and families aren't without somewhere to turn when they have questions or need help. I cannot think of a better way to honor Steve's memory and I am grateful for the opportunity every day.

Meet Sarah Kilch Gaffney

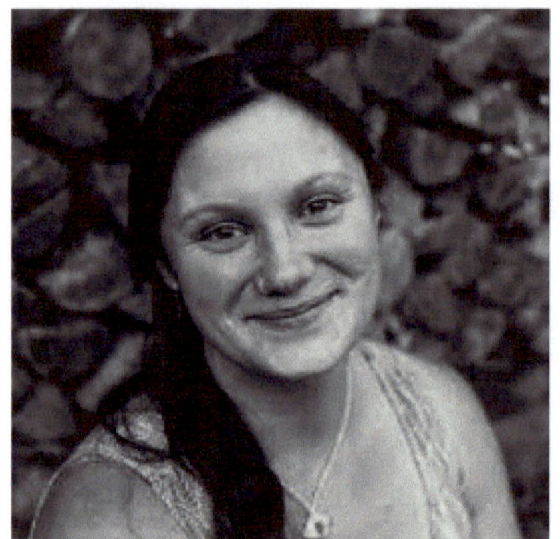

Sarah Kilch Gaffney is a writer, brain injury advocate, and homemade caramel aficionado. You can visit BIAA-ME's website at www.biausa.org/maine and you can find her writing at www.sarahkilchgaffney.com.

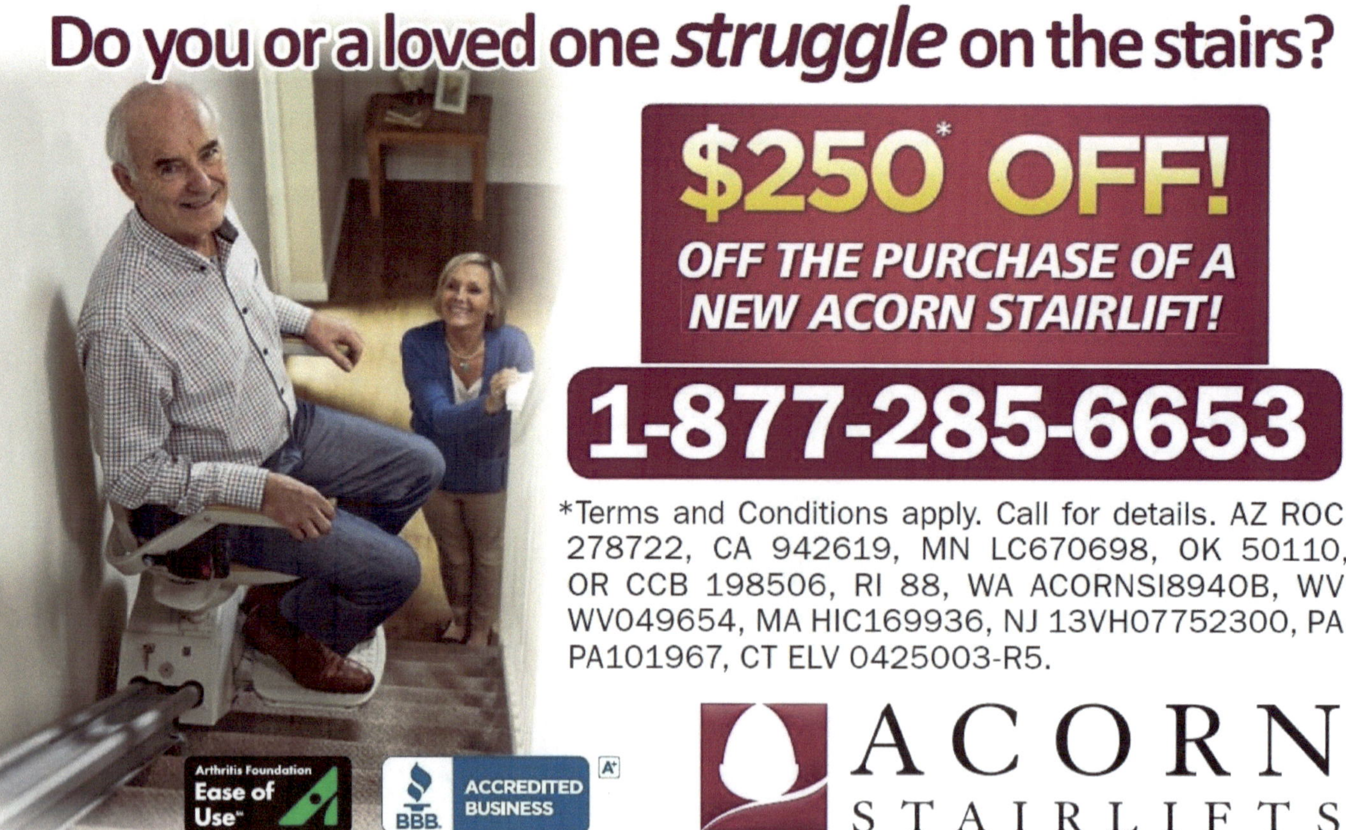

News & Views

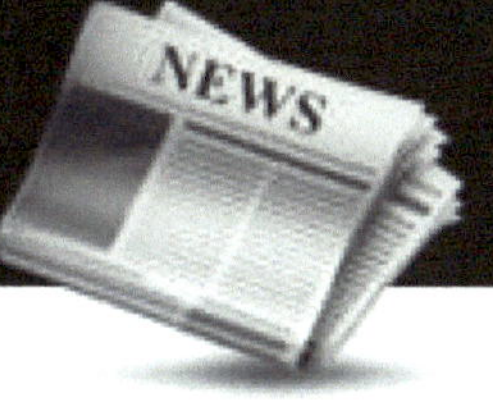

This three-year anniversary issue of HOPE Magazine is our largest issue to date. The stories you have just read are nothing short of inspirational. While going through the process of laying out each issue, I marvel at the true courage of the human spirit.

From rural Maine to Salt Lake City, Utah, the stories shared in our March issue show clearly that brain injury knows no geographic boundaries. Additionally, our Young People's Section reminds us all that anyone, anywhere, and at any age can become part of the brain injury community.

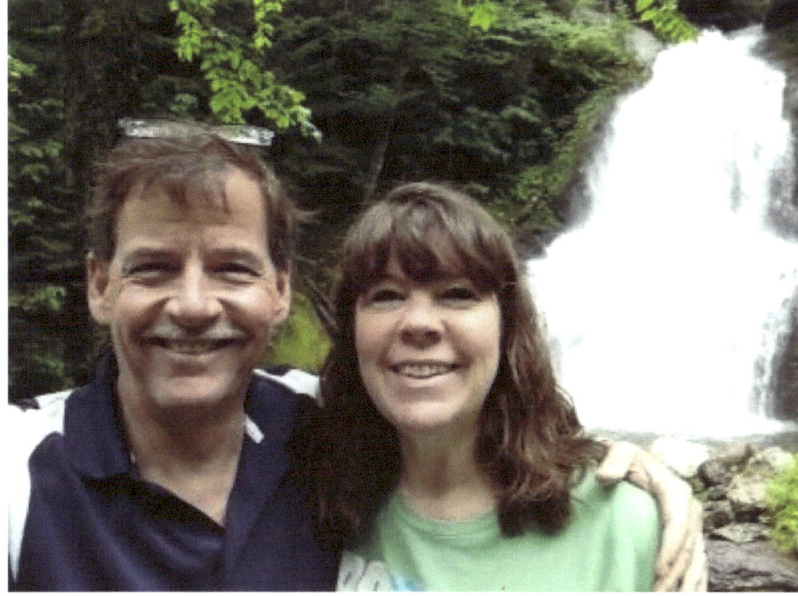

There is an understandable heavy emphasis on brain injury awareness this month. Statewide and nationwide organizations use this month to help educate those unfamiliar with both the prevalence of brain injury, as well as the realities of life after brain injury.

As March comes to a close, we will continue our ongoing advocacy work. I encourage those able to look for *"teaching moments,"* those seemingly random opportunities where brain injury becomes part of the conversation.

Until next month,

~David & Sarah